# How to Help Your
# Loved One Recover from
# Agoraphobia

# How to Help Your Loved One Recover from Agoraphobia

Karen P. Williams

New Horizon Press
Far Hills, New Jersey

Requests for permission should be addressed to:
New Horizon Press
P.O. Box 669
Far Hills, NJ 07931

Williams, Karen P.
    How to Help Your Loved One Recover from Agoraphobia

ISBN: 0-88282-123-7
New Horizon Press

Manufactured in the U.S.A.

1997  1996  1995  1994  1993  /  5  4  3  2  1

*To my wonderful husband, Ed, and my*
*loving family, who have always supported me 100%, and*

*in memory of*

*Dr. Arthur B. Hardy*
*(1913–1991)*

*a very special man who dedicated his life*
*to helping others in need*

*Author's Note*

I would like to express my thanks and gratitude to the following people who have enabled me to complete this book: to my husband for his patience, understanding, encouragement, and unwavering support; to the late Dr. Arthur B. Hardy for his collaboration and many years of dedication to those who suffer from agoraphobia and panic disorder, and to his wife Crucita for all her assistance; to Dr. John E. Leman for his professional contributions and for helping me recover and giving me the opportunity to be involved in the Terrap program; to Sharon Dowdall, R.N., M.F.C.C., who showed me a better way; to Bud Gardner for being the teacher that he is; to Carol O'Hara for her enthusiasm and guidance, which started me on the "write" path; to Duane Newcomb for his editorial assistance and advice; to the numerous Terrap centers, to Mary Ann Miller and Agoraphobics in Motion (AIM), and the many others who graciously participated in my research survey; and to the numerous fellow sufferers and their families who graciously spoke with me of living with and recovering from agoraphobia and panic disorder—your contributions were beyond measure. Without all of you it could not have been done.

All matters regarding personal health require medical supervision. A professional psychotherapist, medical doctor, or other health care professional is an essential member of the recovery support network of anyone who seeks to overcome agoraphobia and panic disorder. The ideas, suggestions, and procedures contained in this book are not intended as a substitute for professional assistance.

The names, circumstances, and other identifying characteristics of individuals, couples, and families mentioned in this book have been changed to protect their privacy.

# Contents

# My Journey from Despair to Recovery

*"You can do anything that you set your mind to accomplish."*
*—Dr. Wayne W. Dyer, Your Erroneous Zones*

I went from being vice president and marketing/sales manager of a credit bureau—one who traveled extensively throughout my local county—to being totally housebound, unable even to drive a car. And it all began suddenly, the result of agoraphobia and panic disorder.

One day, while driving on the freeway to make an out-of-town business call, I had my first panic attack. The sun was shining. It was a beautiful morning—the kind that makes you feel great to be alive. This was a trip I was not unused to, for I had traveled it many times before. Not wanting to sit behind a desk for eight hours every day, I enjoyed being able venture out of the office. Little did I know when I headed out on this spring morning that my life as a normal human being would begin to deteriorate.

Three-fourths of the way to my destination, without warning, I began to feel strange. My hands became cold and clammy. They felt awkward on the steering wheel. I looked around, frightened. The inside of the car seemed to surround me and I felt closed in. My breathing became very short and rapid. There just didn't seem to be enough oxygen. Gasping for air, I felt my heart pounding so hard I felt as if it would pop right out of my chest like a Jack-in-the-box. At the same time my stomach clenched. A fear I had never felt before overwhelmed my whole being. "Do I pull over and stop?" "Do I try to make it to the next town?" My thoughts raced back and forth. My mind was in a complete state of confusion. I rolled the window down, trying to get air. My awareness was suddenly awakened to things I had never paid much attention to before. Noticing all of the cars around me, I realized if I could not maintain my control, I would be in serious trouble.

"Only a few more minutes before I reach the turnoff," I thought. It seemed like an eternity, but I made it. I wasn't sure what had happened to me, but one thing I was sure of was I didn't like it. Fortunately the rest of the day seemed to go pretty normally and I soon pushed my bad experience to the back of my mind.

However, as the weeks passed, these attacks became more frequent. Soon they weren't confined to when I was driving. They started happening at other times, too.

This was getting serious. At first I thought it was just work-related. Then I began having these feelings at other places, too—when I was in the grocery store, at the hairdressers having my hair cut, riding in an elevator, or in crowded places. Shopping alone had always been great relaxation for me, and browsing through the stores at the mall was one of my favorite pastimes. But as much as I had once enjoyed this, I now even started having panic attacks there. Overwhelmed by a growing fear, I decided to just not to go anymore.

Soon my attacks affected my social life with my husband. Ed and I bowled in an evening league which I had very much enjoyed, but even this was becoming unpleasant. Instead of looking forward to our night out bowling, I began to dread it because I was now having panic attacks there, too. What on earth was my life coming to?

Both my work and my personal life were now greatly affected. Plus, I had a new symptom to add to the list that seemed more devastating than all the others: instant diarrhea. When the panic came, I would get terrible stomach cramps and would have to find a restroom quick—or else!

Over the next few months my doctor prescribed a variety of tranquilizers, but not only did they not kelp, they made things worse. As a result, I decided to live with the anxiety rather than live in a tranquilized fog.

Some months passed. As they did, my condition grew even worse. I lived with terrible anxiety. The only way I could keep from having attacks was to stay home, where I felt safe. So unless I had to go to the office, I usually stayed in the safety of my house. According to my doctor, there was nothing physically wrong with me. Thus, I became resigned to the fact I probably had a mental problem and must have been going crazy.

Then one day while cleaning the house, I had the television on and overheard three women discussing panic attacks. I sat down and listened, amazed at the familiarity of what they were saying. As each told her individual story, I listened intently. They were describing what had happened to them, but they were also describing what was happening to me. There was a name for what I had: *agoraphobia*. And these women had become afflicted with agoraphobia because of what they called *panic attacks*.

However, I soon discovered that knowing about the disorder did not make it go away. And since I did not know where to turn for help, it also did not make things any better. Finally I decided the only thing left to do was to go to my doctor and tell him what I thought I had. To my dismay, by the time I had built up enough courage to do this, he had retired. I felt abandoned: Why hadn't he mentioned he was going to do this? I had always felt a sort of camaraderie with him, and now he was gone.

Right back where I started, I still didn't know what to do. My panic attacks were now regular events. Avoiding the places they were occurring was threatening my job and all other aspects of my life. I tried visiting another doctor, but to no avail. Not knowing where to turn, I lived with it as best I could.

One day while out making a business call, I happened to see a flier in a little cafe. It had *agoraphobia* printed at the top in big letters. To my amazement it was an advertisement about a support group for people with agoraphobia. On it was a phone number and a date of the next meeting, but it was an old flier and the date had passed. I wrote down the number anyway, thinking I might at least check into it.

Afraid to call and not wanting anyone to know I had the disorder, I kept the number in my purse for a couple of months. When I did get up my nerve—this person wouldn't know who I was over the phone anyway—I discovered the support group had disbanded. Randa de Lorme, the woman who started the group, said people with agoraphobia did not like leaving their homes; therefore, not enough people came to the meetings. However, since she herself had the disorder and had done a lot of research on it, she said she would be glad to meet with me and tell me whatever I wanted to know.

Reluctantly, I stepped outside my safe domain and met her at a local restaurant a few blocks from home. I had a panic attack while waiting for her to arrive and was just getting ready to head out the restaurant door when in she came. My anxiety must have been apparent, for she immediately walked up and asked if I was Karen Williams.

I suggested a table by the door—in case I needed to make a quick getaway. As we sat down, I found myself revealing for the first time to someone other than my husband my well hidden secret: I had agoraphobia. The noise in the restaurant was deafening. I felt as though I could hear everyone's conversation at each individual table. My heart was pounding, for my anxiety was close to panic level, but I figured I should stick it out as long as I could.

Randa told me how she had recovered from the disorder by gradually exposing herself to anxiety-provoking situations, by taking one day at a time, and by the help and support of her husband. She left with me a folder filled with information about the disorder.

For the next few days I did nothing but read up on agoraphobia and panic attacks. I discovered I was not alone in my suffering. Millions of others had the same problem.

Randa was now busy running her own business and living her life to its fullest, so other than talking to her on the phone a few times, I did not see her again. But the information she gave me was a step on my road to recovery.

Although I now knew a lot about the disorder but still did not know where to turn for help, I eventually resigned from my position at the credit bureau and was on my way to becoming completely housebound. I had the knowledge about what should be done but did not know how to apply it, so at that time it was not really of much use. It is not just enough to know something; one must take that knowledge and put it to use in order to help oneself.

Then one day my husband decided I needed to get out of the house, so he talked me into going with him to visit our friends John and Sue. Reluctantly, I ventured out of my safe domain.

While we were there, I discovered that Sue, for personal reasons, had been going to group therapy sessions for quite sometime. Her group therapist had recommended she attend a speech given by a lady named Sharen Dowdall, who was a therapist and a biofeedback specialist.

For the next year I went to Ms. Dowdall. Although she helped me with many areas of my life, I still had diarrhea and could not seem to completely get over my agoraphobia and panic attacks.

She was not a doctor; she could prescribe no medication for my diarrhea and anxiety disorder. Therefore, I decided it was time for me to try to find a family physician who might know about the disorder and could help me.

Rereading all the information on agoraphobia and panic attacks that Randa de Lorme had given me, I saw the name *Terrap* mentioned. Thinking back, I remembered Randa saying she had heard about a Terrap program in Menlo Park, California, but had never attended. Until I saw the name again and remembered her mentioning it, I had not considered Terrap, for Menlo Park was too far away for me. Not exactly sure what Terrap was but knowing it had something to do with these disorders, I looked it up in my local telephone directory. To my surprise there it was: *Terrap, Sacramento, California.* There was an office right in the next town. Why I hadn't discovered it sooner I'll never know. Maybe I just wasn't ready.

I called Terrap and found the psychologist, Dr. John E. Leman, very kind and understanding. He told me of a good family physician familiar with the disorder, giving me the name of a Dr. Reilly in Fair Oaks, California, a town not too far from where I lived. A man familiar with how people with this disorder think, Dr. Leman said that if I did not like this doctor, I could call him back and he would be glad to refer me to another.

Dr. Reilly was exactly the person I had been looking for. In September 1985 I attended my first Terrap meeting. And with the help of this understanding doctor and a good phobia treatment program to guide me, seven years after I had my first panic attack, and with my husband by my side for support, I began my journey on the road to recovery.

# Why a Recovery Book Involving the Agoraphobic's Family?

*"We cannot prevent birds from flying over our head, but we can prevent them from building nests in our hair."*

—*Chinese proverb*

For the families of many agoraphobics, there are many months or years of not knowing what is wrong with their loved one. Then at long last the sufferer's problem has a name: agoraphobia with panic disorder. While this knowledge provides family members some relief, they still undoubtedly feel distraught, frustrated, and discouraged because they want to help but don't know how. Almost everything they've tried doesn't work. It seems as though they often say or do the wrong thing. And as their well-meaning attempts are either ineffective or rejected, they begin to feel helpless.

As time passes, most sufferers and their families find agoraphobia and panic disorder more and more difficult to cope with. Yet everyone is so focused on the family member who is ill (which is only natural), including the sufferer him- or herself, nobody realizes or even cares about the burden on the other family members. And no one addresses how the disorder is affecting the family as a whole.

Emotional ailments like agoraphobia with panic disorder can often be more disrupting than a physical illness. Most families find themselves totally unprepared for the major adjustments they must make in their lives because of this disorder. It has a radiating effect on all the people who love and care about the sufferer, especially those who live with the person. The illness can also disrupt the entire household routine. And if the disorder has become chronic and ongoing, this not only affects how family members interact with one another, but how they interact with other people in general.

There are three to five million victims of agoraphobia and panic attacks. The number of immediate relatives (spouses and children) whose lives are affected by their close association with one who suffers is an astounding five to eight million people—not to mention other relatives, close friends, and business associates.

As one who suffered from agoraphobia and panic disorder, I realized no one can suffer from these types of anxiety disorders without involving their family. Everyone is affected to some degree.

Unfortunately, I discovered that few doctors or therapists understand the familial nature of the problem. Thus, like the one who suffers, the people closely associated with this person receive little or no help from anyone, and more than likely will be left to cope as best they can. Again, like the sufferer, more often than not these relatives will also feel as if they are the only ones in the world who have this problem intruding into their lives.

It is important for families to realize that there is no magic pill that will instantly eliminate agoraphobia and panic disorder. It will take a lot of hard work and patience on your part to help the person recover. By the same token, the sufferer needs to realize that he or she will get better but must work to accomplish recovery.

The demands of being a good support person require great patience, courage, and determination. It is not an easy task; it can be difficult and overwhelming at times. But for those of you who give wholehearted support, there are also great rewards. It is heartening to watch someone you care for who has been suffering grow and change and know you can share in the success because you are an important part of that recovery.

Although there is no way to foresee every obstacle one might encounter, there are answers to many of the problems that accompany living with and/or supporting a person suffering from this type of disorder. Support people need to build a support network and learn how they and the sufferer can work together to overcome the problem through good negotiation and communication skills. You also need to know what to look for in a treatment program and the qualities a good recovery therapist or doctor should have.

Dr. David H. Barlow, Professor of Psychology at the State University of New York at Albany and co-director for the Phobia and Anxiety Disorders Clinic in Albany, found through his research that when spouses were included as co-therapists, more than 90 percent of agoraphobic patients were much improved at the end of treatment and continued to improve at follow-up. In fact, results were much more favorable at the four- to nine-year follow-up review than those of agoraphobics treated more intensively but without spouses.

Other relatives, and even friends, also make good support people. Dr. Barlow says, "Oftentimes, for middle aged or older women, we found an adult child, such as an adult daughter, is very useful. Other times we found that a close friend makes a good support person."

I had the honor of collaborating with the late Dr. Arthur B. Hardy, psychiatrist and founder of the Terrap (Territorial Apprehension) Program, which has phobia and anxiety disorder treatment programs in many locations throughout the United States. Dr. Hardy passed away in October 1991. A pioneer and foremost leading expert in this field, Dr. Hardy was one of the first physicians in the United States to treat these disorders. He began the first program in America for the treatment of agoraphobia and was a founding board member of the Anxiety Disorder Association of America (formerly known as the Phobia Society of America).

In addition to my several years of research and the expertise of Dr. Hardy, I consulted other experts in the field. With my experiences, from having been a sufferer, a support person, and a paraprofessional, the experiences of other sufferers and their families, plus the knowledge I attained from Dr. Hardy and the other experts, I believe this book is the most comprehensive guide to supported recovery.

Whether you are the sufferer's spouse, parent, sibling, or other relative, or even a close friend, the approaches and techniques covered in this book will make the recovery process easier for you and the sufferer. Although professional help is important, you will learn ways to play an essential part in the sufferer's recovery.

# Anxiety, Panic Disorders, and Agoraphobia

*"This is, I think, very much the Age of Anxiety, the age of the neurosis, because along with so much that weighs on our minds there is perhaps even more that grates on our nerves."*

*—Louis Kronenberger*

In order to live with and help a sufferer recover, you need to understand the nature of anxiety, panic disorder, and agoraphobia. Knowledge is power, and education is the first step to becoming a good recovery support person.

## THE NATURE OF ANXIETY

Anxiety is a state of apprehension, a distress of the mind. An example is being concerned about a possible future event, the uneasiness you might have over its outcome—even if this event is an eagerly awaited one. Anxiety can also be the uneasy feeling you have of being powerless and unable to cope with threatening events. These anxious happenings—often accompanied by physical tension—can come from one's *internal* thoughts (which sometimes stem from the imagination) or from one's *external* environment.

*Chapter 1*

### Anxiety vs. Fear

The American Psychiatric Association points out that *anxiety,* in reference to certain mental illnesses, refers to an unpleasant, over-riding mental tension that has no apparent identifiable cause. *Fear,* on the other hand, causes mental tension due to a specific, external reason, such as when your car skids out of control.

Like anxiety, fear comes in many forms and can be aroused by *external* danger or *internal* thoughts. The physical symptoms of fear are a manifestation of the body's preparation for "fight or flight"—an inborn survival instinct. Anxiety seems to arise from the apprehension of something unpleasant happening in the *future.* Unlike fear, it does not appear to occur because of any detectable cause, thus adding the element of the unknown. The mind alerts the body of danger, activating the same physical responses as with fear, yet psychologically the experience doesn't seem to make any sense.

Everyone experiences some anxiety. Under the proper circumstances, anxiety can be beneficial. A good example of this is the type of anxiety some people feel before taking a test or giving a speech. This type of anxiety can lead to proper preparation and high performance.

Some people even seek out anxiety-provoking circumstances: sky divers, race car drivers, and stuntmen, for instance. Many people also pay millions of dollars each year to feel *secondhand anxiety* through watching a suspenseful movie or a dangerous sporting event.

### Normal vs. Abnormal Anxiety

The intensity of anxiety can range from a very mild feeling to a full-blown, no-holds-barred anxiety attack. When anxiety becomes persistent and out of proportion to the circumstances, however, it is *abnormal* anxiety. At this point a sufferer needs help to overcome the reaction. Still, it's important to note that the person who suffers from this type of anxiety is *not* abnormal; it is the anxiety itself that is abnormal.

### The Three Factors in Anxiety

Within anxiety there are *physical, mental,* and *behavioral* factors. When someone is anxious, he or she feels the effect of all three of these elements at the same time. Understanding these factors will help you to better understand the natural progression of agoraphobia and panic disorder.

### The Physical Factor

For the most part, people's emotions are "felt" by their bodies, and in severe anxiety such feelings virtually involve the whole body. Some of the physiological sensations anxiety causes may include a rapid pounding of the heart, a rise in blood pressure, tense muscles, rapid and difficult breathing, trembling, queasiness, perspiration, urges to urinate or have a bowel movement, a dry mouth, sensitivity to one's surroundings, and even nausea.

Along with these physical sensations, the body chemistry changes. The increased rate and strength of the heartbeat cause oxygen to be pumped at a faster pace. In turn, the spleen contracts, releasing stored red blood cells to carry this oxygen. Sugar stored in the liver is released for use in the muscles. And adrenaline is secreted by the adrenal glands. The flow of adrenaline into the blood stream causes the body to have some of the physical symptoms mentioned. These changes, most of which are internal, all happen in a matter of minutes after one becomes anxious.

*Why the body responds as it does.* The nervous system is comprised of *voluntary* and *autonomic* (or involuntary) nervous systems. We control the voluntary nervous system by such actions as moving our legs to walk or raising our arms to comb our hair. In comparison, the autonomic nervous system has two branches that run automatically and cannot be directly controlled. When we are relaxed, not being stimulated, the parasympathetic branch regulates our bodily functions. Thus we feel calm and laid-back. When we are stimulated, the other branch, the sympathetic system, takes over. It increases our breathing and heart rate, raises our blood pressure, causes us to perspire, makes our muscles tense, and so on. This is the system that reacts when we feel anxiety. When we're no longer anxious, the parasympathetic system calms us down.

The feeling of fear usually stimulates the autonomic nervous system of people who suffer from anxiety disorders such as agoraphobia and panic attacks. Thus their reaction becomes one of anxiety and panic.

### The Mental Factor

The mental factor in anxiety is the anxious thoughts produced and affected by a person's particular state of mind. For instance, anxious thoughts might make people feel on edge or irritable, make their imaginations run rampant, or leave them with the sudden inability to concentrate or sleep.

Psychological stress plays a big role in this element of anxiety. It has recently been recognized that psychological ailments such as agoraphobia and panic disorder may be an outcome of cumulative stress. It seems stress has the greatest impact on the weakest point in a person's system.

Stress comes from inside people and is mainly determined by the meaning people place on particular events in their own lives and environment. As a result, whether people experience stress and anxiety is determined by their own interpretation of life's events. Major life changes such as death of a spouse, divorce, injury, illness, family disagreements, or financial problems can cause stress. People can also find themselves at risk by occurrences that they see as happy events—getting married, having a baby, a job promotion. Experts believe that every significant event or change in a person's life, whether it be good or bad, can cause stress.

### The Behavioral Factor

When people suffer from anxiety, it also has an effect on how they behave. For instance, anxiety sabotages a person's ability to perform certain tasks. It might also lead a person to avoid certain daily activities and circumstances, creating what is called *avoidance behavior*. Thus, the behavioral factor in anxiety is the result of behavior created from a sufferer's reaction to the physical and mental factors. For someone to recover from an anxiety disorder, it is necessary to intervene in all three areas.

## Other Causes of Anxiety: Illness and Medication

Although uncommon, some medical illnesses can produce anxiety, including hormonal disorders such as hyperthyroidism, cardiovascular and respiratory problems, premenstrual syndrome, and menopause, as well as blood disorders, diabetes, and sometimes allergies. Rarely is anxiety their only symptom, however.

Certain medications, both over-the-counter and prescribed, can also cause anxiety. These include thyroid medications used in high doses, asthma and antispasmodic medications, diet pills, cold medicines, and amphetamines. Sometimes antidepressants used to reduce panic attacks can induce anxiety, as can the discontinuation of drugs like sleeping pills, certain tranquilizers, and some blood pressure medicines.

Medical conditions—either illness- or substance-based—that cause symptoms of anxiety but in which the anxiety abates when the medical condition is treated, were recently recognized officially as *organic anxiety disorder.*

Some dietary substances can also heighten anxiety. (These will be discussed in Chapter 11.)

# TYPES OF ANXIETY-RELATED PROBLEMS

The American Psychiatric Association has established a criteria for diagnosing specific anxiety disorders. This criteria is listed in the widely used *Diagnostic and Statistical Manual of Mental Disorders,* referred to as DSM-III-R. The disorders defined are Panic Disorder, Agoraphobia With and Without Panic Attacks, Social Phobia, Simple Phobia, Generalized Anxiety Disorder, Obsessive–Compulsive Disorder, Post-Traumatic Stress Disorder, and Organic Anxiety Disorder. Since some of these disorders coexist with agoraphobia and/or panic disorder, it's important to know the nature of these ailments.

### Social Phobia

People with social phobias have irrational fear of their activities being watched by others, such as fear of signing a personal check, eating a meal in public, or—the most common—public speaking. It is a form of performance anxiety except in that symptoms go well beyond the usual nervousness. Social phobias often develop after puberty and decline after age thirty. A person can suffer from one or more. Men and women suffer from it equally. Some people suffer from social phobia along with their agoraphobia.

## Simple Phobia

Some people have an irrational fear of specific objects, such as animals like mice, snakes, and dogs; or situations, like flying and heights. If the object or situation is one commonly found in everyday life, the disability can be severe. If it's one that doesn't appear very often, it doesn't seriously impact behavior. Simple phobias that develop during childhood usually disappear eventually. In adults, simple phobias rarely go away without treatment.

## Generalized Anxiety Disorder

The main characteristic of Generalized Anxiety Disorder (GAD) is persistent and unrealistic worry that lasts six months or longer and involves two or more distinct personal life situations, such as one's career, health, or finances. Money concerns after a job loss is a realistic concern and would not be a sign. Chronic and excessive worry about events that are not likely to happen would be. Victims of GAD experience a variety of physical and emotional difficulties, and this ailment can coexist with panic disorder, depression, and alcoholism.

## Obsessive–Compulsive Disorder

This disorder is characterized by thoughts or obsessions that invade consciousness, recurring or persisting about certain situations, objects, or places. To relieve their anxiety or reduce the persistent thoughts, sufferers develop time-consuming routines or compulsions and superstitious behavior patterns. For example, feelings of contamination, resulting in repeated washing of hands.

Some agoraphobics suffer from a mild case of obsessive–compulsive disorder, which is often present before they develop agoraphobia.

### Post-Traumatic Stress Disorder

PTSD begins in response to a severe physical or mental trauma—such as rape, fire, flood, airplane crash, military combat, and so on—usually within a few weeks of the incident. Some people merely need to witness an event to become afflicted. Victims continually relive the traumatic event or suffer from general emotional numbness. Symptoms include nightmares and flashbacks, withdrawal from family and friends, sudden unprovoked anger, concentration problems, and insomnia. People often recover without treatment—usually in a matter of months. However, those who are continually troubled for months or years need treatment.

## PANIC DISORDER

The main characteristic of panic disorder is a sudden overwhelming anxiety and fear that occurs without warning and for no apparent reason. Often, this is also accompanied by a feeling of intense fear that one is dying or going crazy. It is also characterized by the sudden onset of any of the following physical symptoms: shortness of breath, fear of losing control, heart palpitations, hot flashes or cold chills, lightheadedness, sweaty palms, perspiration, tingling sensations, chest pains, feelings of being smothered or choking, abdominal distress, diarrhea, nausea, trembling, and feelings of unreality. Almost all victims feel tense muscles and changes in heart rate—some even have others such as blurred vision—but few experience all the symptoms.

In a full-blown panic attack at least four of these symptoms will be present; two or three would be characterized as a *limited-symptom attack*. The attack will reach an intense symptomatic peak within the first ten minutes, then taper off in an hour or less. Although uncommon, in some cases it can return in waves, lasting up to two hours.

*Dan, a teenager, was sitting near the top row of the bleachers with his friends in a school assembly when his heart began to pound. Says Dan, "I was overwhelmed by fear. I wanted to get up and leave, but I felt trapped because there were rows and rows of kids seated in front of me."*

# Chapter 1

*Two months went by without Dan having another anxiety attack. Then one afternoon a friend offered him a ride. "I'd only been in the back seat of his car a few minutes when that awful feeling suddenly hit again. My heart started to race, my hands got cold and clammy, and I began to feel kind of spacey." Dan was so frightened of this feeling happening again that from then on he refused to ride anywhere with his friends.*

*Sharon was in her mid-twenties when she had her first panic experience. "I remember standing in line at the grocery store when suddenly I began to feel strangely unreal. A feeling of panic welled up inside me. I had the urge to run out of the store. By the time I got to my car, the feeling had subsided." Several days later panic struck again when Sharon was in line at K-Mart. "An awful sensation that something terrible was going to happen came over me. All I could think about was getting home as fast as I could." Terrified of the panic experiences, Sharon started to avoid any place where she had to stand in line—grocery stores, banks, department stores.*

The average age at which this type of panic disorder strikes is the late teens to mid-twenties. It is uncommon for it to begin before the age of twelve, although Dr. Hardy treated a child as young as four. It also rarely begins after age forty. However, we have treated senior citizens. Approximately 75 percent of sufferers are women, although this seems to be changing as more men now come for treatment.

The initial panic attack usually occurs after a significant stressful event—for instance, an altercation with a spouse, the birth of a child, an illness, or a job change. Some can also begin with a traumatic experience, as they did for Rita, a middle-aged woman whose attacks started after an automobile accident.

While not common, some first attacks have been drug-induced from using LSD, cocaine, marijuana, and other panic-causing substances. James, for example, who grew up in the sixties, had his first panic attack while getting high on marijuana. Once panic attacks begin, regardless of their origin, the attacks tend to take on a chronic life of their own.

## The Biological Roots of Panic Disorder

Over the past decade the focus has shifted somewhat to include a biological component.

Large amounts of sodium lactate in the blood have been found by some researchers to increase nervous reactivity in panic attack victims. (Sodium lactate is a normal byproduct derived when muscle cells convert sugar into energy.) Thus, using an infusion of sodium lactate into the bloodstream, researchers at Washington University found that panic disorder patients experienced a sharp increase in blood flow to the temporal lobes of the brain—the same areas affected by the normal anxiety that non-panic volunteers felt in a previous study in which anxiety reactions were induced using mild shock.

Researchers also noticed that in an area of the brain known as the parahippocampal gyrus, the blood flow on the right side of the gyrus of individuals who suffered panic attacks was found to be much higher than on the left—thus appearing to distinguish panic attack sufferers from other people.

In another study researchers targeted an area called the locus ceruleus, a small nucleus located in the pons of the brain stem. They found stimulation of this area with certain drugs triggers panic disorder. They also found that panic attacks could be blocked with drugs that inhibit activity in this area of the brain. Researchers then hypostatized that in people who have anxiety attacks, this area of the brain might stimulate easier, reaching higher levels of activity, and thus be more susceptible to anxiety attacks than in people who don't have these attacks.

Many health care professionals believe anxiety that has a strong biological component will not respond well to psychological treatment alone. Nonetheless, it's been found that these sufferers, like all others, can improve their condition by changing their lifestyles, reducing stress, and improving their physical well-being.

## The Diagnosis and Progression of Panic Disorder

Panic disorder is diagnosed when an individual has had four or more unexpected panic attacks in one month or one panic attack followed by four weeks of persistent worry about having another. On the average, attacks occur two to four times per week. Between panic attacks there is a tendency for a sufferer to become apprehensive and fearful of having another one, thus developing *anticipatory anxiety.*

According to the American Psychiatric Association's *Diagnosis and Treatment of Anxiety Disorders: A Physicians Handbook,* panic disorder may progress through the following stages:

**Stage 1** Limited symptom attacks
**Stage 2** Panic Attacks
**Stage 3** Hypochondriasis
**Stage 4** Limited phobic avoidance
**Stage 5** Extensive phobic avoidance
**Stage 6** Secondary depression

(Although there may be variations, half of all cases start at Stage 1, the other half start at Stage 2.)

The disorder may evolve rapidly (over days or weeks) or slowly (over months or years). If the unexpected anxiety attacks are frequent and intense, the patient can progress rapidly through all of the stages. If the attacks become milder, the patient may remain at the existing stage and not progress further until the attacks again increase in frequency or severity.

## Medical Ailments That Coexist with Panic Disorder

There are some medical ailments that a few professionals believe coexist with panic disorder. These ailments produce some of the same physical sensations as the disorder. Other professionals believe that disorders like these can coexist yet still be unrelated, each ailment being a disorder within itself that needs to be treated. Such disorders can include hypoglycemia (low blood sugar), mitral valve prolapse (a benign arrhythmia of the heart), and inner ear disorder. Irritable bowel disorder—a chronic gastrointestinal condition where one experiences abdominal discomfort and pain along with changes in bowel habits with no gastrointestinal disease present—may be another; however, researchers hypothesize that this illness is, for some, a symptom of panic disorder.

## Panic and Anxiety Disorders and Heredity

Most researchers feel that to some degree anxiety and panic disorders are hereditary. However, researchers differ as to heredity's role. In the Washington University study mentioned earlier, the preliminary findings of an "extended" study showed that panic disorder itself may involve a hypersensitivity of the septo-hippocampal region of the brain—the part of the brain that matches and compares input information from one's environment, memory, and body. Evidence suggests that this hypersensitivity is transmitted through the chromosomes from generation to generation.

Other research findings indicate that people do not inherit the anxiety disorder; they inherit the predisposition to be "overly anxious." This makes them susceptible to having anxiety problems. In other words, they are born with an "excitable personality type" (which will be discussed more later) common among anxiety disorder sufferers. After that, it depends on individuals' particular environment and upbringing.

According to Dr. Hardy, if one parent has an "excitable personality type," at least one of the children will inherit this characteristic. If both parents do, most of the children will have this trait to some degree.

Dr. Hardy generally gave his patients a family tree (see Figures 1 and 2) and asks them to place an apple on the tree for each relative who had an anxiety problem. Figure 1 is an example of this family tree completed by a patient. Here most of the anxiety problems occur on the mother's side. The other tree (Figure 2) is provided to help you trace the sufferer's background.

Every child is different. One child with a wet diaper, for example, might lay in the crib indefinitely without being bothered, while another might cry the very minute the diaper gets wet. Another child could sleep through all kinds of noise, while still another would wake at the slightest sound. Researchers have discovered that even at birth children already possess a host of built-in reactions as part of

Chapter 1

Figure 1. The Family Tree. This tree was completed by a sufferer of agoraphobia and panic attacks. The apple on each branch represents a relative who has or might have had anxiety, fears, shyness, agoraphobia, or a drug or alcohol problem or been hospitalized for nerves. The letter within the apple represents the following: A=agoraphobia; D=drugs or alcohol; F=fears; N=nerves; S=shyness; X=anxiety.

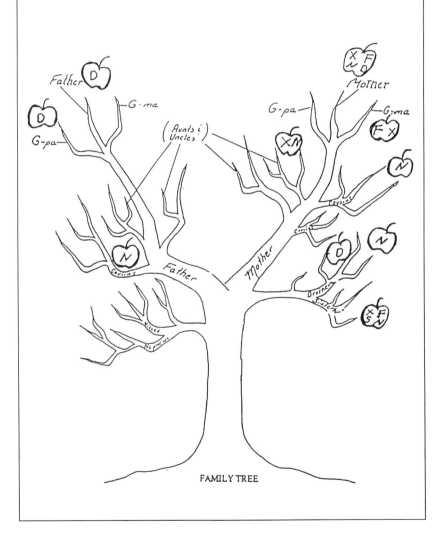

FAMILY TREE

**Figure 2. Your Family Tree.** To trace your family tree, place an apple on each branch that represents a relative who has or might have had anxiety, fears, shyness, agoraphobia, or a drug or alcohol problem or been hospitalized for nerves. Use the key from Figure 1.

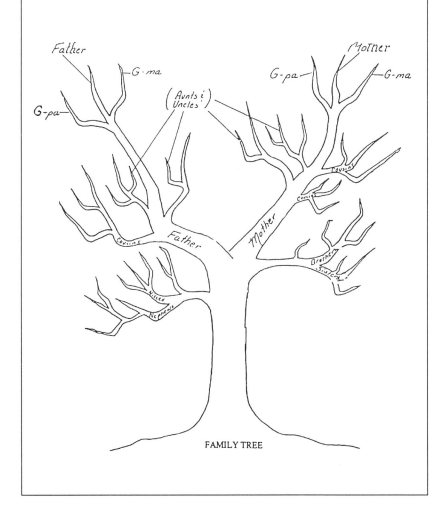

their inherited biological make-up. Thus certain characteristics that appear very early on in life appear to be inborn.

Recognizing a child's behavioral characteristics early can allow parents to provide children who have inherited "excitable personalities" with the proper environment and attitude.

Although studies are still ongoing, it appears that panic disorder and agoraphobia run in families. Figure 3, provided by the National Institute of Mental Health, shows the "schematic evolution of spontaneous panic attacks."

## AGORAPHOBIA

Agoraphobia is the fear of being in particular places or situations that are away from one's area of security, that is, one's safe place or safe person. The disorder usually begins full-blown with a panic attack while victims are away from home—on the way to work, standing in line in the grocery store, or driving on the

**Figure 3. Schematic Evolution of Spontaneous Panic Attacks.**

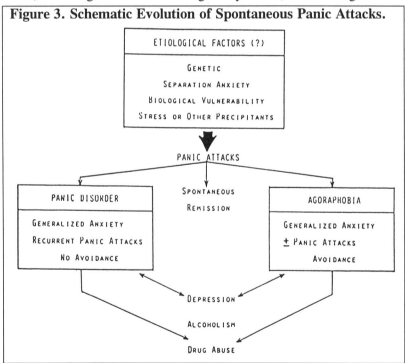

freeway. There is no "common" place or circumstance where an attack will happen, but attacks usually occur away from home or apart from someone the sufferer depends upon.

Along with the panic attack and its debilitating physical symptoms, agoraphobia victims feel an internal sensation of impending doom. They fear their anxiety reaction will continue to get worse until they finally "go to pieces" or end up screaming and hysterical in front of others. They especially fear loss of control or making fools of themselves in public.

## The Anxiety Scale

The symptoms of anxiety that agoraphobics feel during a panic attack almost always appear in the same order. The anxiety scale below (Figure 4) shows the succession of physical symptoms they experience. (It is based on a scale of 1 to 10, with 10 being complete panic.) These symptoms involve both the mind (which includes the emotions) and the body; the two cannot be separated.

| Figure 4. The Anxiety Scale. | |
|---|---|
| 10 panic—disoriented, spacey, detached, frantic, hysterical; numbness, strange sensations | *Area of nonfunctioning* |
| 9 dizziness, nausea, diarrhea, visual distortions, numbness, some hysteria, fear of losing control | |
| 8 stiff neck, headache, feelings of doom | |
| 7 tight chest, hyperventilation | |
| 6 lump in throat, muscle tension | *Area of decreased ability to function* |
| 5 dry mouth, need to escape | |
| 4 shaky legs, tremors | |
| 3 rapid heartbeat, tremors, muscle tension | *Area of continued ability to function* |
| 2 sweaty palms, warm all over | |
| 1 butterflies in stomache | |

When sufferers retreat, usually to their homes, the panic symptoms subside. Other than the memory of extreme discomfort, sufferers quickly return to their original state, although many do feel "drained" for some time afterward. Escaping to home teaches sufferers that their houses are secure, safe places. Home then becomes their "area of security."

The attacks also become associated with the situations or places where they occurred—a learning process known as classical conditioning. Sufferers developed a "learned response" in reaction to their fear. First people have a fearful reaction to one particular store, bridge, or roadway, then their reaction generalizes to all stores, bridges, or roadways.

As time goes on, the sufferers' fears become more widespread and more pronounced. In my case the fear reaction started on the freeway, then eventually spread to stores. Gradually sufferers withdraw from all situations they expect will cause the uncomfortable unpleasant feelings of anxiety and the awful physical sensations that accompany the attacks. Agoraphobia is developing.

### The Stimulus Response

Have you ever stuck yourself with a needle while sewing on a button? If so, your automatic reaction was probably to jump. The *stimulus* here would be the pinprick and the jump would be the *response*. But a stimulus does not have to be a physical one; it could be a mental stimulus, such as a negative remark that creates a hurt feeling.

Stimulus ——————➤ (creates) ——————➤ Response

A person's response is usually in proportion to the stimulus that created it. However, a small stimulus sometimes produces a large response. That is what happens in agoraphobia. Sometimes the stimulus is so small, the person doesn't even recognize that it exists. To this person, it seems as if such a reaction came out of the blue. Waiting in line at the grocery store, for example, might provoke anyone just a little, thereby being a small stimulus. Yet for an agoraphobic this small stimulus creates a large response, one that is way out of proportion to the circumstances. The response is what creates the physiological reactions shown earlier in the anxiety scale (Figure 4).

small stimulus  ——————➤ (creates) ——————➤ BIG RESPONSE

When one becomes stimulated enough to have a response, it always takes time for one's body to return to normal. During this period, there are several peaks of anxious feelings, decreasing in waves, before the body normalizes. With each peak the anxiety decreases. However, there must be no further stimulus, and people must have the ability and the opportunity to discharge their tension in order to recover normally. If the stimulus is repeated too soon, or if releasing their tension is inhibited, the tension remains.

When complete recovery is not achieved after each stimulus, people soon become increasingly sensitive. Thus, with each new stimulus their tension increases. Then, any stimulus, no matter how small, increases the sufferers' level of tension, prolonging their recovery time and leading them to react out of proportion to everything.

## The Principle of Sensitization

You also need to understand the principle of sensitization. The agoraphobic in the grocery store was sensitized to a particular stimulus: lines. Everyone experiences sensitization. Just watch someone eat a lemon and see what happens to *your* mouth—it's so sensitized to how a lemon tastes that it can almost taste the sourness. We are also sensitized to pleasant stimuli, such as the aroma of apple pie baking in the oven. Just thinking about how good it smells can make your mouth water, which just goes to prove that a *thought*, as well as an object or a circumstance, can serve as a stimulus.

## Agoraphobia's Natural Progression

Some people develop comfortable ways to live with their disorder, like sitting by the door or in an aisle seat at the movies or church so they can make a quick getaway.

Bill owns a very successful chain of sporting good stores and feels he must stay involved with local sporting events and activities. He liked to attend local basketball games, for example, but to do so gave him panic attacks. So he made some compensations: "I found if

I sit on the bottom bleacher, near the door, I am able to sit through the whole game. I know I can leave if I have to, so I don't feel trapped." Bill has a mild case of agoraphobia. He and others like him can continue working and shopping but otherwise don't venture too far from home.

In more moderate cases, sufferers begin to avoid certain situations or places (restaurants, elevators, movie theaters, and public transportation) or circumstances (crowds and baseball games). They can handle certain things away from home, although they have some discomfort, and are only partially restricted.

June, for instance, loved to shop at a particular department store but was unable to ride escalators or elevators. Since ladies' clothes were located on the second floor, June would call ahead and make arrangements for an employee to bring clothes downstairs. This helped but kept her from facing her fears. June was also an avid golfer and could play as long as her husband played with her. She led a fairly normal life, but she had not been on a vacation in many years and was unable to go to shows, attend church, or drive on the freeway alone.

Others develop severe agoraphobia, as I did. They eventually become afraid of so many situations and places that they literally develop a phobia of the world—a world that, unless the agoraphobics seek help, gets smaller and smaller until it leaves them totally housebound unless accompanied by their "safe" person. I started out like Bill, then my fears progressed to where I was similar to June. Finally I ended up with a severe case. I was fortunate, however, in that my disability didn't continue getting worse for years and years. I was eventually able to find proper help—but I have known phobics who have been housebound for many years.

Many sufferers, whether they have a mild, moderate, or severe case, wait as long as ten years before seeking treatment. However, research shows—and I am living proof—that over time the disorder will worsen if help is not sought. Dr. Hardy found that some sufferers who avoid facing their problem eventually develop anxieties even in their "safe" places, becoming unable to be left alone.

. . .

### Worrying about the What-If's

The main component of agoraphobia becomes the underlying syndrome "phobophobia," or the fear of the fear itself. When the sufferer contemplates exposure to anxiety-producing situations, the "what-if's" develop. "What if I have an attack?" "What if I have to leave in a hurry and can't get out of here?" "What if I'm stuck in traffic?" "What if I get too far away from home?" Sufferers make no distinction between thoughts and actual events. Therefore, they react to such thoughts as if they represent unavoidable danger or harm.

The what-if's lead sufferers to become chronic worriers. Their anxiety begins to build up in advance of being in a certain place or situation, and thus anticipatory anxiety and phobic avoidance develop.

### Alibi-itis

What Dr. Hardy referred to as "alibi-itis" also occurs. "To avoid surprises that might endanger their own security," he said, "sufferers begin to make excuses. The alibis start. They become artists at inventing reasons for avoiding anything that has the remote chance of causing trouble. As the affliction progresses, the excuses become better and more believable."

### The If-Only's

Regretting the disorder, agoraphobics often develop "if-only" thinking. I was a good example of doing this. I used to say, "If only my parents had taught me to be more independent, I never would have turned out this way." Then, because I always wanted to be what I thought people wanted me to be, I thought, "If only I could have been more myself." And I regretted, "If only I could have really told people what I thought." For sufferers, if-only thinking arouses real and painful emotional reactions.

### Agoraphobia's Fluctuating Nature

Agoraphobia is not a logical disorder. It is a disorder born of emotions. Feelings of phobic anxiety can change from day to day or week to week. Some days, regardless of circumstances, victims have very few episodes of phobic anxiety, while on others, anxiety is quite high. Attacks do not follow a straight line.

It is important to realize that sufferers are neither insane nor incompetent. Even during a panic attack, suffers are sometimes capable of being logical and taking appropriate action if the situation warrants it. However, this does not mean they are faking their fears and anxiety the rest of the time.

## Other Problems Agoraphobia Creates

Agoraphobia is often compounded by other problems. Agoraphobics are likely to develop depression and fatigue. Some suffer from alcoholism, social phobias, and mild obsessive–compulsive disorders.

### *Depression*

Depression is inevitable for agoraphobics because of the discouraging nature of having such a restrictive disorder and the disintegrating effects it has on the sufferers' relationships with family and friends.

"Can't" has become the main focus of their existence: "I can't go to my kids' soccer game," "I can't have company over," "I can't go out to dinner," "I can't go to church," "I can't go to the grocery store," "I can't drive on the freeway." They are cut off from most pleasurable activities and are often too dysfunctional to perform mundane ones, like grocery shopping. As I did, they often feel guilty for having to lie and make excuses and guilty because their disorder restricts their families' activities.

The first episode of depression sometimes happens within weeks or months of the initial panic attack. This often aggravates the agoraphobia. Crying spells, feeling "blue," or feeling irritable or hopeless are typical. Sufferers may also have difficulty sleeping. Fortunately, depression is not the main problem—the disorder is. Once the disorder is treated, the depression lifts.

·   ·   ·

## Fatigue

Many agoraphobics suffer from exhaustion, because they have sleep problems. Some have a difficult time getting to sleep. Others go to bed early and sleep late, only to retire before noon for a nap. Others wake regularly in the middle of the night, then have trouble falling back to sleep. Then they just can't seem to get going. Getting motivated to overcome the disorder is difficult.

## Alcoholism

According to the Anxiety Disorder Association of America, "Nearly one-third of Americans with an anxiety disorder turn to alcohol for comfort." It temporarily relieves them of their attacks of anxiety. It also dissipates phobic fears more completely than other drugs, such as tranquilizers.

Some individuals believe drinking helps calm them before going out in public. These people usually tend to avoid social events where alcohol is not served. Other sufferers use alcohol in order to go to work, attend school, and even drive a car. One agoraphobic, a big burly fellow, always carried two cans of beer in his coat pocket just to get him through situations he feared. In his case, however, he never opened them—he just used them as a crutch.

However, alcohol can actually contribute to the feeling of loss of control and unusual bodily sensations, thereby exacerbating panic instead of reliving it. Alcohol can also interfere with treatment. Alcohol depresses the central nervous system, thus reducing the effectiveness of exposure treatment. Agoraphobics who consider themselves recovered due to the use of alcohol are also vulnerable to relapse.

## Decreased Sexual Desire

The sex life of the agoraphobic sometimes becomes disrupted and sporadic. However, reports show that 83 percent of agoraphobic men still regularly enjoy sex after the onset of the disorder, as compared to only 60 percent of the women. The disorder can also cause so much frustration, anger, and resentment in a couple's relationship that it has an adverse effect on most of their pleasurable activities—including the desire for sex.

The fatigue that victims experience also accounts for the lack of sexual desire. And the lack of sexual interest from one spouse often becomes regarded as a painful rejection by the other. The longer the disorder persists, the more difficult maintaining a good relationship becomes.

Anxiety, panic disorder, and agoraphobia are all part of the same equation. The more you understand their nature, the more you will be able to help the sufferer recover.

CHAPTER TWO

# Understanding the
# Agoraphobic Personality

*"There is an invisible garment woven around us from our earliest years: it is made of what we eat, the way we walk, the way we greet people, woven of tastes and colors and perfumes which our senses spin in childhood."*

—*Jean Giraudoux*

To fully understand how phobias develop and why the recovery techniques detailed in this book work, it is important to understand the basic characteristics of the agoraphobic personality.

Although no two people are alike, there are certain personality traits that consistently show up in almost all agoraphobics. Research shows that agoraphobics are extremely sensitive and have what Dr. Arthur B. Hardy called an "excitable personality." When stimulated, even mildly, they respond easily and intensely. At the drop of a hat they will cry, feel sad, angry, hurt, or lonely. But they will just as easily feel affectionate.

## THE TOTAL BODY RESPONSE

When people with excitable personalities respond to a stimulus in terms of feelings, they have a total body response. For instance, if the response is sadness, they feel sad all over. A good example is blushing, a body response reddening the face when one's blood vessels dilate in reaction to a stimulus. This is an external reaction; there are many internal physiological responses that cannot be seen. However, as any sufferer will confirm, they can be felt.

The difference between the average person and the agoraphobic is the way they respond to stimuli. The sufferer responds quicker, with stronger emotions, reacting intensely to sensations of touch, taste, smell, sounds, or sight.

When allowed to be themselves, these people are creative, loving, talkative, outgoing, interesting, fun to be with, and often sought after. They have active imaginations and are also intelligent, ethical, and can relate well to others.

Some aspects of this personality trait, however, make life more difficult. Such people are easily upset and tend to be too dramatic, often over exaggerating. They are not only sensitive to their own moods and feelings, but those of others as well. When people with whom they are close are fearful and anxious, they soak these feelings up like a sponge. That's why it's so important that the people they are close to be fairly stable—not nervous, neurotic, or fearful.

## People Pleasers

Another trait sufferers have in common is the need to be all things to all people. Dr. Hardy called them "people pleasers." They are sensitive to what others think of them and go out of their way to accommodate others' wishes instead of satisfying their own. Rather than taking the initiative to do what they'd like to do, they spend their time being over-concerned about what others think, thus feeling self-conscious. They like to avoid conflict and work hard to gain people's approval.

Agoraphobics are also "people pleasers" to ensure they will never be abandoned. Sufferers must cling to others, because they are no longer self-sufficient or independent.

Their sensitivity to what people think usually makes agoraphobics overly afraid of being embarrassed. In their minds, making a fool of themselves in front of others is absolutely forbidden. That's the main reason many keep their disorder hidden. As they often say, "If people really knew, they would think I was nuts." Unfortunately, when they keep their phobia bottled up, it only magnifies these fears and intensifies their anxiety about them.

## Passive–Aggressive

About 20 percent of Dr. Hardy's clients had a tendency toward passive–aggressive personality habits—a serious trait that interferes with recovery. They complained, whined, were stubborn, procrastinated, blamed others, and were angry in general for having their problem—all passive–aggressive symptoms. They also wanted someone to solve their problems for them. Yet they were "people pleasers." Because of their behavior, he said, these sufferers learned they had to become "people pleasers" or the people they were close to might leave them.

## Perfectionism

Another trait most agoraphobics share is that they are perfectionists. They have a tendency to set unrealistically high goals, which they then worry about not being able to meet. They also strive to live up to goals that they have let other people set for them. This leads them into "have-to" thinking: "I have to go to college, because my parents want me to" or "I have to keep the house immaculate, because my husband expects me to." They even try to live up to the goals of people they don't know. For example, while in a restaurant they might think to themselves, "I've ordered this sandwich, now I have to stay here, because the waitress expects me to." Have-to's place the control over their lives outside themselves, creating constant frustration and resentment inside.

## Criticism

Such individuals also go out of their way to avoid being criticized, for criticism might lead to hurt emotions and a feeling of not being wanted. To avoid being criticized, they again strive for perfection and often make larger demands on themselves than necessary.

Criticism is a powerful inhibitor of the free expression of feelings. Often there is or was a member of the sufferer's family with a need to consistently pass judgment on others, including the sufferer, by criticizing. Maybe a parent didn't actually tell a child he or she was dumb but said, "I wish you had your brother's brains. He always gets good grades." This made the child believe he or she was dumb: if the parent said so, it must be true!

Criticism leaves sufferers filled with self-doubt. Thus, they are never quite sure of their own acceptability. They often wonder, "Am I worthy? Am I good enough?" Eager to please, they must always "be nice to everyone" and "look their best," the result being that they tend to please at all costs to avoid being criticized. Sometimes they also internalize the values of the critical person, thereby becoming self-critical and critical of others. When criticized, they tend to react by criticizing and demanding perfection from others. Fortunately, their need for perfection and pleasing others decreases as they begin to recover.

## Inhibition

Like criticism, inhibition is another common denominator. Sufferers become inhibited for a variety of reasons. Most often, somewhere in their lives someone is or was a strong inhibiting force—a person in a position of influence, most often a parent or a spouse who suppresses the child's will to assert his or her impulses and feelings. A perfect example would be a child who is punished for speaking out or acting impulsively, or one who is not allowed to show anger. This creates a self-inflicted inhibition, whereby they believe that they must maintain control of their feelings at all times.

Sufferers also have acquired an inhibiting effect from their culture—a culture, for example, from which they learned to always behave like a "lady" or a "gentlemen." When the sufferers' impulses and feelings are suppressed over a long period of time, they often reoccur when the individual is under stress, which results in anxiety or panic.

Feelings are the energy that motivates people's behavior to do things. This is what leads them to action, which in turn discharges their feelings and releases their tension. If people have inhibitions that block the release of tension, they can have feelings without discharging the tension these feelings create. This leads to problems. As Dr. Hardy explained, "If the energy of feelings cannot find an acceptable outlet for release and inhibition thereby exists, malfunctions of the nervous system can result."

It's extremely difficult for people with excitable personalities to discharge their tensions through normal channels. They are too inhibited to do so. Becoming less inhibited is important for them, for this will release their tension, and released tension will help decrease their sensitivity.

## Separation and Dependency

Although little research has been done, "separation anxiety" in childhood—experiencing anxiety, panic, and other bodily symptoms when separated from a parent—seems to predispose adults to have agoraphobia. It leads to an overdependency trait. Children who are overdependent upon their parents are generally children that are overly fearful. "Separation anxiety" is more than just the fear of being separated from a parent. It is the fear of being separated from the safety a parent provides in particular situations that are anticipated by children as mentally or physically dangerous.

While the dependency pattern begins to appear in early infancy, most children are able to move, little by little, away from areas of security. Slowly, they develop a feeling of confidence about themselves, and as they do, they acquire the emotional ability to cope with their own fears and injuries. Some children, however, have temperaments or upbringings that lead them to continue to cling to their parents and their homes as safe havens. These children often go on to develop anxiety in adulthood when becoming separated from a "safe" place or "safe" person.

## Insecurity

Abandonment caused by a divorce or death, along with neglect, rejection, and even physical or sexual abuse, can also produce insecurity in children—as can growing up in a family where one or both parents are alcoholic. During the time children are most dependent upon their parents—from infancy to approximately age five—any situation that fosters insecurity can lead to excessive dependency. Whether children later develop agoraphobia or other anxiety disorders depends upon the way in which they react to the events in their lives and the degree of insecurity they develop.

Some agoraphobics were anxious and tense as children, due to a constant feeling of insecurity. They suffered from fear of the dark and nightmares; some feared becoming ill or dying. These children usually had over-protective parents who had an especially cautious view of the world. Their parents continually and repeatedly warned them about danger: "Be careful not to get too cold." "Don't get to close to Johnny or you'll catch something." "Watch out or you'll hurt yourself." Such warnings communicated to their children that the world was a dangerous place. When the children were sick or hurt, the parents reacted as if it was a major catastrophe. These children modeled themselves after their parents and developed an over-cautious attitude not only about the world but minor illnesses or other problems.

Children like this often grow up with a tendency to worry too much. They become overly concerned about their own safety, so they limit taking risks or exploring new places and things.

On the other hand, some believe that parents who overreact in the opposite way—pushing their children to be "heroes"—can produce the same results. In situations where there are logical reasons for these children to be fearful, these parents insist, "Don't be afraid" or "Don't be such a baby." These children become afraid to show or even feel fear, because if they do their parents will scold or reject them. Unfortunately, when reality is traumatic these children become more frightened instead of less. Their fearfulness then spreads to other areas in their lives.

### Behavioral Conditioning

As discussed, conditioning is nothing more than a procedure that changes people's behavior patterns. With classical conditioning, the combining of two different stimuli induces a learned behavior pattern. But there are two other types of conditioning that can affect behavior traits and lead individuals to develop agoraphobia.

There is *operant conditioning,* whereby particular consequences are brought together that either increase or decrease the rate or intensity of a desired activity. Reinforcing a particular activity with rewards, for example, would make the activity stronger. A child whose parents reward him or her with praise and encouragement for completing a difficult task—whether done perfectly or not—is a good example. The parents' reward gives the child a feeling of accomplishment and motivates him or her to take risks, thereby trying other difficult things. Operant conditioning also works well when used to motivate a sufferer during recovery.

However, operant conditioning could also be induced by punishment, which would decrease an activity. A child who is continually punished for expressing thoughts becomes an adult who holds everything inside. Such a person often develops agoraphobia with panic disorder.

Unlike the first two types of conditioning, which require repetition to instill the behavior patterns, the other conditioning, known as "modeling," requires only observation. For example, the type of children mentioned earlier were insecure, because their parent(s) had an overly cautious view of the world, which led them to model themselves after their parents' fearful attitudes and behavior.

Along with their genetically inherited tendencies, sufferers have also been variously conditioned throughout their lives to develop the behavior patterns that make them vulnerable to agoraphobia. Although conditioning causes sufferers to develop certain behavior patterns, it can also help them to unlearn these same patterns through what is known as "behavior modification."

## Accepting the Sufferer's Behavior

It's important to remember, throughout recovery, that the habits and behavior patterns of the sufferer were developed over a lifetime and therefore cannot be changed overnight. It is vital that you accept the sufferer for the type of person he or she is at this moment. Focus on his or her good qualities, not the bad. Recognize that the agoraphobic has become sensitized to a variety of things and is therefore supersensitive. This is not his or her fault but the fault of a lifetime of poor conditioning. Make a special effort to help the sufferer understand how he or she became so sensitive. This is the first step sufferers can take in learning how to desensitize themselves. And this is the first step you can take in helping them to do so.

If you can help the sufferer think of him- or herself as a person who has been conditioned, this person will not feel so guilty or desperate for having the disorder—or for being the type of person he or she is. This is something that is temporarily out of his or her control.

## Learning about One's Own Disorder

You now understand more about the sufferer, his or her disorder, and why this person might have developed it; however, it is important that the sufferer also become educated about his or her own disorder and the type of personality characteristics that lead to it. Whatever treatment program this person chooses to follow, education should always play a vital part.

I have found that some relatives fear that if their loved one concentrates on his or her problem, it will cause their disorder to increase, making matters worse. But nothing but positive benefits come from a sufferer's self-education about the disorder. Experts have found that learning about one's own disorder reassures the afflicted person, improves the outcome of his or her recovery, and enhances this person's cooperation in the recovery process.

When you finish reading these chapters, have your afflicted loved one read them also. The two of you (and any other relatives interested in being a member of the support team) can then discuss the information. When you discuss this information, it not only helps to better understand the problem, it gets the disorder out into the open so you can start talking about it. This communication—the sharing of each other's thoughts, feelings, views, and ideas about the disorder—helps you both understand one another better, and this in turn helps you successfully work together on recovery.

# The Most Effective Recovery Techniques

*"A good beginning makes a good ending."*

*—English proverb*

There are three main areas of intervention that are useful in treating agoraphobia with panic disorder. The first is cognitive/behavior-oriented treatment, the second is psychotherapy, and the third is medication. Some sufferers require all three simultaneously in order to recover, while others need only one or two. For example, some individuals need to use medication to bring down their anxiety level enough to successfully employ the cognitive/behavior-oriented treatment techniques. Others might also have personal problems that interfere in their recovery. As a result, they also need psychotherapy from an anxiety disorder specialist. Some sufferers, however, need just one of these interventions. When this is the case, it is usually the cognitive/behavior-oriented treatment process.

## BEHAVIOR-ORIENTED TREATMENT

Behavior-oriented treatment is considered to be the most effective treatment for agoraphobia, especially when combined with cognitive therapy. When used together with other recovery techniques, the results are usually very good.

Since a phobic reaction is a conditioned response—developed from a learned habit—it is not only changeable, but erasable. In the beginning sufferers become sensitized to a stimulus. Therefore, they must become *de*sensitized to this stimulus in order to recover.

In experiments with cats, psychologist Dr. Joseph Wolpe conditioned the animals to develop an avoidance reaction to a compartment of particular size, shape, and color. First the cat was placed in a compartment and shocked, causing it to avoid the compartment. The researchers then used the cat's drive for food along with the pleasure the cat experienced while eating it to overcome the cat's avoidance reaction to similar compartments.

Then, in a succession of similar trials, this process was repeated until the cat entered the actual compartment in which it had originally received the shock—the cat had been reconditioned to reverse the avoidance reaction. Dr. Wolpe called this conditioning process "systematic desensitization."

Wolpe and other researchers then applied this technique to human phobias. If someone was afraid of mice, for instance, treatment would start by having this person think about the word *mouse*. Next this person would be asked to imagine the word *mouse* written on a paper, then to imagine a picture of a mouse, then to imagine a mouse in a glass case, then to imagine they are holding a mouse, and so on.

Between each step, researchers had the subjects do deep-relaxation exercises to counteract the anxiety that each individual step would arouse—similar to food counteracting the cat's anxiety. When subjects were able to handle one step without experiencing any anxiety, they moved on to another step. Each step took a week and sometimes longer, depending on the individual.

Ultimately, "imaginal" desensitization progressed to real-life exposure, or in-vivo desensitization. This became the treatment of choice.

The sufferers' avoidance response is the main key to successfully reducing their fears. Therefore, desensitization, when done correctly, is the road to recovery.

# COGNITIVE THERAPY

Cognitive therapy essentially involves people's thoughts and feelings about their disorder. Cognitive therapy helps sufferers learn to analyze and control their various thought patterns and assumptions, separating the realistic from the unrealistic. Much of the anxiety sufferers experience can be contributed to their fallacious beliefs—erroneous ideas about themselves and about the "fearsome" world they live in. Along with creating anxiety, these habitual defeatist ideas can lead to poor performance, anger, frustration, and resentment in the sufferer.

The first step in cognitive therapy is for sufferers to recognize the false beliefs they have been carrying around in their minds. The next is for them to define what these beliefs actually mean, thereby being more objective about them. This procedure helps sufferers to identify the mistaken concepts they have about phobic situations and to realize these concepts are only thoughts, not fact or reality. Once this is accomplished, they test their mistaken beliefs against real-life situations to see how unrealistic and absurd they actually are. The final step is for them to revise and correct these fallacious beliefs.

This is mostly done through internal self-talk, which will be discussed later. When sufferers approach or anticipate anxiety-producing situations, they mentally say negative things to themselves about what they believe will happen, statements such as "I'll faint in the middle of the store" or "I'll be trapped in the elevator." Using cognitive therapy, these negative statements are revised in one's thoughts and changed into positive statements: "The reality is I won't faint" or "The reality is people rarely get trapped in elevators." These statements are then modified from the imagination into actual reality situations by a technique known as "reality testing" (also be discussed later).

Cognitive therapy is used in combination with other treatment techniques. It is a vital recovery tool, one that is very powerful when combined with the desensitization process.

It's important to note that various forms of behavior and relaxation therapy go by different names, such as contextual therapy (which is the use of imaginal and in-vivo desensitization combined) and autogenic training (a relaxation technique that uses both body and mind). However, they are all similar in technique and purpose.

## RELAXATION AS AN ANXIETY-REDUCTION TOOL

Fear of a panic attack causes victims to become mentally anxious and in turn to physically tense their muscles as a way of maintaining control. When this happens their ability to think logically diminishes, because they are so anxious.

Relaxation skills help sufferers face the panic-producing stimuli by enabling them to regain control of their bodies during an anxiety attack. Relaxation therapy is based on the concept that it is not possible for people to be both tense and relaxed at the same time.

The parasympathetic nervous system's response can be willfully activated to stop and reverse the body's emergency response—the one that's triggered by an anxiety or panic attack. The sufferer's unconscious mind has been typically held accountable for whether the body is tense or calm. But every sufferer's body actually has a built-in control switch that allows him or her to calm the sympathetic (emergency) response, thereby relaxing the major muscles of the body and significantly reducing their anxiety.

There are a variety of methods used to teach sufferers to relax at will, the most common being breathing exercises, tension-relaxation (muscle tensing preceded by muscle relaxing), static-relaxation, emotional-relaxation (imagery), cue-controlled deep muscle relaxation, meditation, and biofeedback.

### Anxious Breathing

The way people feel is closely related to the way they breathe. For example, slow diaphragmatic breathing is associated with calmness, whereas fast and shallow breathing is related to anxiety. Improper breathing can lead to over twenty-five symptoms of anxiety, faintness, feelings of unreality, shortness of breath, and heart palpitations to name a few.

The sufferers' patterns of breathing are always involved in their anxiety and panic. In relaxed and natural breathing, which comes from the diaphragm, people breathe in and out the nose, taking in slow, rhythmic breaths. This natural rhythm of breathing is disrupted when people become anxious or distressed.

These sufferers override the autonomic nervous system, exerting voluntary control over their breathing. When they are anxious they tend to take shallow rapid breaths. They also tend to hold their breath or over-breathe, hyperventilating. Many sufferers also tend to breathe from the upper chest, sometimes drawing air in and out through the mouth.

Although the sufferers' breathing patterns are part of the problem, they can also be part of the solution. People can actually change how they feel by voluntarily controlling the way they breathe. Thus, learning to breathe naturally from the abdomen (diaphragm), along with avoiding tendencies to over-breathe or hold one's breath, is one of the basic recovery techniques.

## Relaxing the Muscles

When sufferers prevent the discharge of their muscular tension or hold in feelings of any intensity that have been aroused, their muscles remain tense. This leads victims to suffer from what is called *residual tension*. Residual tension, along with the victim's anxiety and phobias, can produce symptoms such as indigestion, insomnia, headaches, backaches, and irritation.

The more muscle tension sufferers can eliminate, the more they can totally relax their bodies and their minds and the fewer symptoms of anxiety they will have.

I am going to briefly describe four exercises I learned while going through the Terrap program. Many phobia and anxiety programs and self-help books use these relaxation techniques or very similar ones—many also make available to the consumer relaxation exercises on cassette tapes.

Sufferers can do any of these exercises either sitting in a chair, on the couch, lying in bed, or even on the floor.

●   ●   ●

# Chapter 3

## Tension Relaxation

In tension relaxation, sufferers are taught to first tense, then relax, the muscles.

Lie on the bed, and start with the feet: curl the toes and hold them until some tension develops. Then let the tension go and relax. Feel this tension drain from the feet. Next, move up to the calf muscles: tighten them, hold it, then relax and feel the tension drain away. Then progress to the thighs, stomach, back muscles, and so on all the way up to the muscles of the face.

Sufferers usually start with tension-relaxation exercises. It's easier for them to recognize what relaxation feels like when they start by tightening their muscles. Thus sufferers should practice this exercise until they develop some skill at it before moving on to other muscle relaxing procedures.

## Static Relaxation

Static relaxation uses the same procedure as in tension relaxation, working the way up the body starting with the feet. This time directly relax each group of muscles without tensing them first. The goal is to be able to relax the muscles without having to tighten them first.

Direct attention to the feet and allow them to completely relax until all the tension is drained out and the feet feel heavy. Move to the lower legs and do the same thing. Slowly progress up the body, relaxing the different muscle groups.

## Emotional Relaxation

In emotional relaxation, sufferers use their imagination to help them relax. This is basically a light form of self-hypnosis. This procedure can be done by itself, but should also be used immediately following tension relaxation and static relaxation exercises. Emotional relaxation will add to these two processes by freeing sufferers from their anxious thoughts, giving them a broader sense of relaxation.

Sufferers imagine themselves in a very peaceful setting, a place where they can feel comfortable. This peaceful scene can be an imaginary one or a real place they have been to before, for example, a serine lake amid the pine trees, a babbling mountain brook, a warm sunny beach, or a cozy fireside on a rainy evening.

In this special place, they are to notice particular things they would like to find or see there—trees, water, or animals such as birds or deer. Visualizing every detail helps the scene absorb full attention, deepening the state of relaxation. They must hear the sounds and smell the aroma of the air, even imagine touching things to feel their texture. If this special place is at the beach—as mine was—they would picture the waves rolling into shore and the sun glistening off the water. They would hear the sea gulls and the roar of the ocean. They would also feel the warmth of the sun and texture of the sand between their toes. The idea is for them to thoroughly enjoy being there enough to allow themselves to feel totally relaxed.

The aim of this exercise is not only for victims to be able to relax, it is for them to learn how to create a *safe place within their minds*. This safe place is extremely important, for it allows sufferers to control their levels of stress. With frequent practice this safe place can become so solidly established in sufferers' minds that they can return to it at a moment's notice. Suffers can use it to remove themselves from stressful situations without really having to physically leave them.

### Cue-Controlled Deep Muscle Relaxation

The sufferer's aim is to become mentally aware of what muscle tension feels like in specific areas of the body, then to willfully release that tension. Cue-controlled deep muscle relaxation is an exercise recommended by psychologist R. Reid Wilson in his book *Don't Panic: Taking Control of Anxiety Attacks*. This exercise is done in three stages.

Sufferers are asked at specific intervals during the exercise to repeat a cue word, such as *relax*. The physical relaxation of the muscles then becomes associated with that cue word, creating new circuits between the sufferer's brain and muscles. The goal is for muscles to automatically release at the mention of the cue word.

Stage one is similar to tension relaxation in that one tenses and relaxes the various muscles. Stage two is similar to static relaxation, and stage three (done the last few minutes) is similar to emotional relaxation in that one goes into one's safe place.

## Time Involvement

These exercises themselves take only about twenty to twenty-five minutes. However, at first they should be repeated a minimum of twenty minutes at least once a day (twice or three times if possible) over a period of several weeks or longer.

The past habit of tensing the muscles must be replaced with a new *good* habit—relaxing the muscles. In order to accomplish this, it is necessary for sufferers to practice regularly. Frequency produces desired results.

*Daily meditation* has been found to reduce chronic anxiety. Meditation on a regular basis can also help people who suffer from anxiety disorders to restructure their thought patterns more productively, breaking up obsessive thinking.

*Biofeedback* can help people learn to relax. It can also help them learn to control their anxious reactions. Learning relaxation techniques to calm down when anxiety levels begin to rise can help people recover without the use of drugs. Biofeedback is a way to give people ongoing information regarding the degree of tension or relaxation in their own bodies, making them more conscious that relaxation is occurring. Thus it's good for those who have difficulty learning to relax.

When considering biofeedback, sufferers should look for a biofeedback specialist who has expertise in agoraphobia and panic disorder. This specialist should also be a health care professional trained to listen to sufferers and help them understand any feelings that might surface once they begin to relax.

## Resistance to Relaxation

Relaxation cannot be forced. It must be allowed to develop gradually. Some individuals have a difficult time learning to relax, especially in the beginning. Relaxation implies letting go or losing control, which agoraphobics are afraid to do. Even though they don't realize it, keeping their muscles tense is a way for them to hold in their feelings. In these cases, extra help is often needed.

# THE DESENSITIZATION PROCESS

The desensitization process is divided into three segments: imaginal desensitization, visual desensitization, and in-vivo desensitization.

To use the desensitization process sufferers must first identify the stimuli that set off their anxiety reactions. This is done by making a list of everything that causes the person to have an anxiety reaction. These fears are rated from the mildest to the one that produces the most anxiety, and this is known as the sufferer's "hierarchy" of fears.

## Imaginal Desensitization

Imaginal desensitization is almost always used first, since the sufferers' first area of avoidance begins in their minds. In imaginal desensitization, using their "hierarchy" of fears, sufferers start with their least bothersome fear first, and use their minds to imagine they are in this anxiety-provoking situation. They stay in this imaginal situation until they feel slightly uncomfortable—a #3 level on the anxiety scale (Figure 4). Although mildly anxious, the sufferers picture themselves as they would like to feel in this situation—seeing themselves remaining calm. Then they dismiss this thought and allow themselves to completely relax by retreating to a place where they normally feel safe and at ease—using their mind's safe place. When they have entirely recovered from any anxiety the imaginary situation caused, they repeat the process. The idea is to continually repeat this process until the thought of the particular anxiety-producing situation causes little or no anxiety. The more the sufferer practices, the better the exercise will eventually work in real-life situations.

These steps are what Dr. Hardy called the "five Rs": *react, retreat, relax, recover,* and *repeat.*

## Visual Desensitization

This is the next step in the desensitization process. Sufferers use the same fearful situations from their "hierarchies," but instead of imagining these situations, they look at pictures (photographs, slides, or videos) of these things. Photographs can be obtained, for instance, by cutting out pictures from magazines; for example, pictures of crowds, freeways, people seated in movie theaters (these are easier to find than you may think). Many recovery programs also provide slides or videos of common fearful situations.

The five Rs are again used. Starting with their least fear first, sufferers look at a picture of the fearful situation until they have a *reaction*—again only to a mildly uncomfortable #3 anxiety level. Then they *retreat* by turning the picture over or walking away from it, distracting their mind in the process. Next they *relax* and allow themselves to completely *recover*. They *repeat* this process until they can look at the picture and feel little or no anxiety.

## In-Vivo Desensitization (Exposure Therapy)

In-vivo desensitization is the most effective of all treatment modalities, especially when preceded by a period of orientation, education, relaxation training, and imaginary and visual desensitization.

The final step in the desensitization process is to approach the fearful situations in-vivo, "in real life." In in-vivo desensitization sufferers use the same stimulus from their hierarchy list, again starting with the least bothersome fear, but they now approach it in real life. The situation always remains strictly a *practice* event, not a *demand* event.

The five Rs are again utilized. Sufferers approach the fearful situation until they have a #3 anxiety level *reaction*. They *retreat* by turning around and either walking away, taking some steps towards the exit, or just standing where they are but facing away.

Repetition is the key to success. The more sufferers repeat the desensitization procedures, the closer they can get to their fearful situations, and the longer they are able to stay in them.

.   .   .

### Desensitization to Bodily Symptoms

I would like to briefly mention a fairly new process, developed by Dr. Barlow and his associates, that is having significant treatment success. (This should be done under the supervision of a trained professional.) Using a modified version of exposure therapy, Dr. Barlow exposes patients to their bodily symptoms while not actually in an anxiety producing situation. He might spin his patient around in a chair until this person felt dizzy, or he might have the patient hyperventilate until this person felt light-headed and tingly all over. Then, adding certain cognitive interventions, Dr. Barlow would help the person become accustomed to feeling that way, thus letting this person know he or she could handle feeling lightheaded or tingly and realize, "I'm not going to die" or "I can handle this."

Here are two desensitization process that are also sometimes used:

*Flooding*

This process is extremely difficult do to without a trained therapist. It requires that sufferers stay in the anxiety-producing situation for long periods of time (generally at least two hours), without retreating, even if their anxiety gets considerably high. The goal is for sufferers to remain with the stimulus until their anxiety dissipates, thus decreasing the ability of the stimulus to cause them anxiety.

*Intensive Therapy*

This process requires that a professional work with one patient eight to ten hours a day, five to seven days a week for up to two weeks, helping this person to face fears and overcome anxious reactions. Although effective, when this treatment is first begun, it can be hard on the sufferer's nerves.

## PSYCHOTHERAPY

Psychotherapy alone will not cure anxiety disorders such as agoraphobia and panic disorder, for the psychoanalytic treatment processes used to treat them are basically the same ones psychologists use to treat other neuroses—delving into the past to find the root of the problem. The psychotherapist employs this insight therapy in order to help victims recognize their repressed emotions, so they can confront these emotions and realize they are not bad. The result is that these patients no longer have to hold such feelings inside. Since this type of psychotherapy is conducted in a therapist's office and does not help sufferers face their anxiety-producing situations, Dr. Hardy believed it to be of limited value.

So why psychotherapy? Psychotherapy helps sufferers who have other personal problems significantly interfering with their treatment; for example, those whose lives are full of personal turmoil or those who feel they themselves interfere with successfully recovering from their disorder. The psychotherapist delves into how such people's past events relate to their present-day functioning.

Group insight psychotherapy, however, was found not to be helpful. When patients continually discuss their fears in front of fellow sufferers, this tends to reinforce the fears of others and lead them to pick up new fears, causing them to avoid the group meetings altogether. Insight therapy seems only to increase the groups fears instead of decrease them.

## THE ROLE OF MEDICATION

The majority of doctors and clinicians who treat these afflictions usually believe it is best to explore natural methods of recovery before trying psychopharmacological agents. Many people can and have recovered without the use of these drugs. Nevertheless, professionals agree that medication can be beneficial in many cases. This is especially true when the sufferers' anxiety and fears so immobilize them that they are unable to carry out the treatment techniques or in cases where bouts of panic are so incapacitating that sufferers are unable to leave the safety of their homes to visit a psychotherapist's office.

Although medication does work, there is no medicine that will "cure" anxiety, agoraphobia, or panic disorder. However certain drugs can be helpful in reducing anxiety and panic attacks, enabling sufferers to confront their phobic situations (as in in-vivo desensitization). These sufferers thereby gain experience with coping skills and a better understanding of their problem—the things that are needed to effect a complete and long-lasting recovery. Once these things are achieved, the medication can be slowly withdrawn. The goal is for medication to get sufferers on an even keel, so they can work to overcome their disorders. Another strong reason for medication use is serious depression existing along with the disorder.

Some drugs reduce or diminish the anticipatory anxiety sufferers feel before going into situations that would ordinarily produce their panic symptoms. Other drugs control the panic itself—some users reporting their panic no longer erupts in phobic situations, even though they expect it to because they are still afraid in these places.

There are several classifications of drugs effective in relieving anxiety and panic attacks. Two are antidepressants—MAO (monoamine oxidase) inhibitors and Tricyclic antidepressants—the others being Bezodiazepines (a fairly new category of drugs), Beta-Blockers, and Buspar (busprione), also new. Each medication has its own advantages and disadvantages. Thus, medically supervised experimentation is required from sufferers to determine which medication and dosage level works best for them. Unfortunately, this is not easy on sufferers, requiring patience and understanding from both them and their families.

More and more evidence suggests that the best results for many sufferers is medication in combination with a comprehensive recovery treatment plan. Nonetheless, experts believe medication usually works better on a temporary basis. As Dr. Hardy said, "Medication may help people take the initial steps necessary to leave their safe place. However, I have found medication offers them only a short-term relief of their symptoms." While it's been reported that 90 percent of people who take medication ultimately reduce or eliminate their panic, those who use it to cover up their symptoms and thereby avoid solving their problems have a high relapse rate when medication is discontinued. They also seldom get well. In a nutshell, medication can be used as a treatment modality, but behavior modification is basically the cure.

## Tricyclic Antidepressants

These drugs are used for the management of panic disorder and panic disorder with agoraphobia. Since these disorders often require months and occasionally years of maintenance drug treatment, physicians usually recommend tricyclic antidepressants first because they can safely be used over a long period. Also, they do not cause physical dependence. There are three tricyclic antidepressants that are found to be effective: Tofranil (imipramine), Norpramin (desipramin), and Pamelor (nortriptyline). Among these three, Tofranil (imipramine) is usually the medication of choice, for it is by far the most studied of all the tricyclic drugs used. While these are "antidepressants," it seems sufferers do not have to be depressed to benefit from their anti-panic effectiveness.

## MAO (Monoamine Oxidase) Inhibitors

These drugs are found to be useful for depression with severe anxiety. They inhibit nerve transmissions in the brain that may cause depression. Of all the anti-panic medications, it's been said that MAO inhibitors may be the most effective, for they are sometimes the only drug to which some people respond. They do, however, limit their user in some areas. It is said that MAO inhibitors must not be combined with certain prescription drugs and some over-the-counter cold remedies. People who take them also should not eat foods that contain the chemical tyramine—found in aged cheeses and a number of other foods—for these foods can cause a severe drug reaction. Once these things are avoided the serious side effects of these drugs are reported to be impressively reduced.

Of the MAO inhibitors used in clinical psychiatry, Nardil (phenelzine) is the only drug to be studied regularly. It seems to be the drug used most often. Compared to Trycyclic antidepressants, MAO inhibitors are said to be easier to tolerate for many users.

### Bensodiazepines

Benzodiazepine tranquilizers are used to treat generalized anxiety disorder and panic. What makes these drugs effective is that they are a central nervous system depressant. The benzodiazepines that are reported to be most useful for panic attacks are Xanax (alprazolam)—which is the most commonly used today—and Clonopin (clonazepam). Benzodiazepines are very effective for some people, stopping panic within the first few days. While they are similar to sedatives such as barbiturates in their affect on users, they have few side effects when compared to tricyclic drugs and MAO inhibitors. The main cause of concern, however, is their ability to cause symptoms of physiological withdrawal when discontinued.

### Beta-Blockers

Beta-blockers can be helpful for sufferers with obvious bodily symptoms such as pounding heart, shakiness, and perspiration. These drugs act to block a major chemical reaction in the body's nervous system. Beta-blockers are sometimes used in combination with bensodiazepines to treat panic attacks. The beta-blocker most often used for panic disorder is Inderal (propranolol). When given in a single dose, this drug can be used to relieve the anxiety some people feel before speaking in public or taking a final exam. Although it can produce some side-effects, it is relatively safe. However, when taken regularly it can cause physical dependence, leading to withdrawal symptoms. To discontinue use, the dosage must be gradually reduced.

### Buspar

Buspar (buspirone) has only been on the market since 1987. While it is used to diminish generalized anxiety, this drug has been found ineffective in reducing panic attacks, both in frequency and intensity. However, Buspar does not cause sedation, nor is it habit forming, which leads many to prefer using it over benzodiazepines to treat anxiety. Since it is a fairly new drug, more studies are needed to completely evaluate its usefulness.

## THE BASICS FOR A SPEEDY RECOVERY

It is impossible to give a definite date when a particular person will recover, but one thing is certain: sufferers never recover until they are ready. (Readiness will be discussed in the following chapter.) Sufferers also never recover until they have the proper treatment. Can anything shorten recovery time? According to Dr. Hardy, the basic steps that must be taken to speed recovery are:

1. Understand the problem via education.
2. Establish a safe place, a safe person, and a loving atmosphere in a secure domain.
3. Learn effective relaxation.
4. Learn to face things in small increments while allowing oneself to retreat.
5. Perform in-vivo (real life) desensitization with help from a support person or therapist or by self-help.
6. Build self-esteem and self-confidence by learning coping and social skills.
7. Learn to understand and express feelings.
8. Learn to solve one's own problems.
9. Take charge of one's own life.

How long it takes sufferers to recover, he found, depends on:

1. the sufferer's understanding of the problem
2. willingness to make efforts
3. readiness to do what is necessary to recover
4. complications in a sufferer's life
5. the ability of the sufferer to solve his or her own problems.

I would like to add one more step to this list:

6. the willingness and ability of the sufferer's family to help this person recover.

Next to the sufferer being ready to get well, this can hasten recovery faster than anything else.

# Determining Whether the Sufferer Is Ready to Recover and Finding a Recovery Program

*"The key to success isn't much good until one discovers the right lock to insert it in."*

—*Chinese epigram*

## READINESS TO RECOVER

It is important to understand whether your afflicted relative is ready to recover. The truth is that sufferers will be ready to recover and accept help only when they are tired of being in the pits. This means that the greatest motivator victims can have is their own suffering.

However, some victims can be so passive that they tend to wait for someone to fix the problem for them, while others are just too embarrassed or ashamed to ask for help. These sufferers may try to hide their problem yet still expect family members to be sensitive to their wants and needs. Relatives can then further complicate the situation by failing to honestly admit the existence of the disorder.

This dilemma, known as the "family myth," can require family members to continuously conspire in order to maintain the fabrication, thereby being just as destructive to recovery as family members who consider the disorder a permanent feature in their lives.

Marriage, in-laws, or other family difficulties and attitudinal problems, along with financial troubles and complications from substance abuse or depression, can seriously interfere with recovery readiness. Dr. Hardy found that even strict religious convictions some sufferers put upon themselves can sometimes interfere.

Readiness to recover basically depends upon how many complications sufferers have in their lives that have a bearing on their condition. In addition, a small percentage of sufferers are hesitant to give up their phobic state, because there are inherent rewards in remaining phobic. These rewards, known as "secondary gains," are the advantages and psychological benefits both the sufferer and the family derive from maintaining the disorder. Besides influencing readiness, they can also slow progress once recovery has begun.

## Personal Factors and Secondary Gains

There are personal factors and secondary gains that keep sufferers from being ready to recover. Often they are deep-rooted issues of which people can be unaware. Since everyone's situation is different, you might even think of some personal issues relating to your own situation that were not included.

### *Secondary Gains*

1. Sufferers find it hard to make changes in their situation because inherently the disorder provides them with attention and support (emotional, financial, or both) or allows them special benefits and advantages they feel they otherwise might not have. For instance, relatives and friends run errands or do chores for them, and they don't have to face many adult responsibilities. Suffers also often find their disorder holds people closer to them, sometimes causing family members to become more cohesive and they fear that recovery will change this family closeness.

Sufferers need to be assured by family and friends that recovery will not change their closeness to them. Sufferers also need to realize how being more responsible for taking care of their own needs will make them feel much better about themselves. Recovery doesn't mean they have to face responsibilities totally alone; others will still be there to help.

2. Sufferers sometimes realize their spouse or parents inherently find security in holding on to them, thus they hold back from recovery so as to not upset the relationship. The spouse or parents can be consciously or unconsciously reaping secondary gains from the sufferer having to be dependent upon them. There may be an inherent fear that if the victim completely recovers, this person will become more independent and eventually leave them.

If the marriage is a "rocky" one, the spouse may very well leave. However, if the marriage is a normal one (with its share of ups and downs), these sufferers need to be assured that when they recover the spouse is not going to leave. That recovery will enhance their relationship because of all the things they will be able to do together. On the other hand, the sufferer's spouse must realize that the only way his or her partner will be held back is if these sufferers are unconsciously cooperating to help maintain this person's secondary gains. They must have more faith in their ailing partner and realize they are doing the person more harm than good by keeping the sufferer dependent.

3. Sufferers find recovery frightening, because recovery requires change. Being unsure of how their lives would change scares them. Hence such people are so fearful of risking change, they find it much easier to accept living with their disorder than to work at overcoming their fears. Thus they adjust their lives accordingly.

Sufferers need reassurance that change will be for the good. They need to be reminded of how much better their lives will be once they have recovered. They need to be told that recovery is worth the effort.

*Personal Factors*

1. The sufferers' problem has isolated them to such a degree that they find themselves unable to handle the everyday dealings that accompany taking charge of their own lives. They want to recover, but they are afraid to do so—either consciously or unconsciously. Their coping skills have diminished due to lack of use, causing them

to lose confidence in their own capabilities. Thus these people fear things like getting a job and earning an income.

Sufferers need to stop thinking so far into the future and realize that recovery is a "one day at a time" process they can take at their own pace. They need assurance that they are not expected to completely recover next month or even next year and that family and friends are there to help them.

2. Many sufferers have such a passive, non-assertive approach to life that they don't realize they are entitled to get more out of life. They have an underlying belief that they don't deserve to recover and thus are unable to grant themselves the right to get well. This is self-punishment.

Sufferers need to realize that they might harbor feelings of guilt for having the disorder. Dr. Hardy believed the sufferers' guilt to be a low-grade fear of retaliation or of some consequence for something they have done or said that is contrary to a significant person's values or rules. These sufferers need to stop living by what others think. They also need to work on their self-esteem.

3. Some sufferers inherently fear freedom. Just as many people are afraid to die, subconsciously such individuals are afraid to live. Freedom calls for them to take risks and to confront their fears and anxieties. Some fear if they were truly free there would be nothing to keep them from going out of control, thereby reacting on their hostile or fearful impulses.

They need to understand that their fear of losing control confuses having freedom with being helpless. They need to realize that the recovery techniques will teach them how to eventually place their trust in themselves, and that the less they fear freedom, the less they will feel helpless and the greater their sense of inner security and safety.

4. Some sufferers use alcohol or tranquilizers on a regular basis to relieve their anxiety. Their self-medicating keeps them from having to face the reality of their disorder. They need to realize that these substances interfere with recovery. They also need to be aware that it could mean they have another problem (a substance abuse problem) to deal with on top of agoraphobia and panic disorder.

5. Sufferers lack motivation because they believe there are no

inherent reasons for them to recover. They will not exert the effort recovery takes because they believe there are no future rewards in recovery, "so why bother to try." Another reason they lack motivation is that recovery could lead them to lose a "secondary gain." Sufferers need to find a reason to get well. They need to realize that "insufficient motivation is the biggest roadblock to recovery."

6. Sufferers do not feel responsible for their problem, often attributing them to the stressful people in their lives, heredity, a bad childhood, an abusive upbringing, and so on. These sufferers must realize that accepting complete responsibility for their own recovery is the most powerful thing they can do for themselves. It's important to note that while taking responsibility does not mean blaming others, it also means not blaming themselves for having the problem.

7. Sufferers unconsciously believe that recovery requires too much work. Already feeling stressed out from the disorder, it seems overwhelming to take on more responsibility and work in order to recover. They can also feel despairing that recovery takes time and is not an overnight process.

These sufferers must replace the negative assumption that recovery requires too much work with the knowledge that they can break recovery down into small steps. That way it doesn't seem so overwhelming.

These issues usually need to be resolved before recovery can be initiated. Unfortunately, some individuals are so determined to keep their disorder that they continually refuse or deliberately ignore all forms of help.

## HELPING THE SUFFERER GET READY TO RECOVER

To help a loved one recover, let them know you have found a way to support them and are willing to devote your time and effort if they are willing devote theirs. Since a sufferer's readiness is all-important, the rest is up to them.

*The most important thing you can do to help a sufferer get ready to recover is to make sure he or she knows that you care.*

Sufferers need to know:

- that you take the problem seriously and you sincerely want to help them overcome the disorder.
- that you will work with the person from the beginning, being there until he or she can manage by him- or herself.
- that you believe the sufferer can recover, even if the sufferer doesn't believe it; that you have faith in the person's ability to recover. Belief is vital.

*The second thing you need to do is to offer the sufferer reasons to recover.*
Stress that:

- He or she will lead a more satisfying life, once recovered.
- He or she has a choice. The person can let this disorder discourage him or her or use it as an opportunity to learn more about him- or herself and what he or she can accomplish in life.
- He or she is a wonderful person. The core of his or her being is not his or her disorder (although at present it might seem like it) but this person's intelligence, competency, dependability, creativity, sensitivity, and likable ways (mention any good quality that comes to mind). His or her fear has become so much a part of him or her that this individual has overlooked or forgotten all of these wonderful qualities inside this person. These qualities have probably been erased by self-doubt, and you would like to see these positive aspects of this person's personality resurface again.
- His or her agoraphobia is a springboard to personal growth. Once this person has recovered, all sorts of possibilities will open up. It is possible not only to take charge of his or her own life, but to grow beyond his or her condition. Just the fact that this individual had this condition and overcame it will give him or her a unique opportunity for personal growth and self-exploration.
- Suggest the person imagine being able to enjoy life every day and have choices, or to imagine being free of worry, fear, and anxiety. That is what recovery is all about.

# WHEN IS IT NECESSARY
# TO SEEK TREATMENT?

Although some sufferers may have periods of temporary improvement, generally agoraphobia and panic disorder get progressively worse when left untreated. Thus, the sooner a sufferer seeks treatment the better.

However, the length of time a sufferer has had the disorder is not a deterrent to recovery. As a matter of fact, Dr. Hardy found that those who have had the disorder the longest often get well the fastest. He believed it was because longtime sufferers are highly motivated, due to being tired of having their condition.

If the disorder is beginning to interfere with the sufferer's daily life, affecting things like social functioning, employment, obtaining an education, or personal relationships, along with affecting the lives of his or her family members, it's time to seek help.

# IS OUTSIDE HELP NEEDED?

The treatment approach one chooses should depend upon the severity of the problem. Experts say if the disorder causes no avoidance or mild avoidance, individuals may not require treatment from a therapist or recovery program. These sufferers may only need self-educational training in anxiety and panic management techniques, combined with clear-cut instructions on how to self-direct their own exposure treatment.

In cases where avoidance tends to be more severe, experts advise using individual therapy from an anxiety disorder specialist, or attending a comprehensive group treatment program specializing in anxiety disorders. It is believed, however, that those who avoid a variety of situations may do well placed in group treatment. As for those who are highly avoidant of just a few situations, the treatment of choice may well depend upon which plan affords them the most adequate practice. If individual therapy, for example, gives someone who has driving problems more opportunity for assisted in-vivo exposure (allowing them individual fieldwork) than a group program might provide, then that may be the best recovery plan. When family members become involved in treatment, however, this affords sufferers the most opportunity to practice, no matter what treatment they choose . . . and for the least amount of cost, as compared to paying for individual exposure treatment.

# LOCATING A GOOD RECOVERY PROGRAM AND THERAPIST

The recovery rate from agoraphobia with panic disorder is high, yet only one out of four people seek help. Of those who do, it is not uncommon for them to have been in other forms of therapy for several years without making significant progress. The reason: The treatment of agoraphobia and panic disorder are "specialty" fields, requiring an experienced health care professional trained to treat these disorders specifically.

The acting director of the National Institute of Mental Health, Dr. Alan I. Leshner, Ph.D., reports, "With appropriate treatment, as many as 90 percent of people with panic disorder can be relieved of the repeated and unexpected bouts of overwhelming fear that characterize this disorder."

## Deciding on a Method of Treatment

Just as there are a variety of treatment techniques for agoraphobia and panic disorder that are similar in nature, there are a variety of ways treatment can be structured.

Here are some things to consider before deciding on which method to use:

1. What does the sufferer (and you, if you're going to be involved) want to get out of the recovery treatment program?

2. How much time is involved in using this method?

3. How much effort will it take on the sufferer's part (and yours) to be successful?

4. How much will it cost, compared to how much are you willing to spend?

The following is a review of the various ways treatment can be structured. (Medication can be used in combination with any of these treatments.)

### *Individual Therapy with an Anxiety Disorder Specialist*

The majority of therapists who specialize in anxiety disorders such as agoraphobia and panic disorder offer individual therapy treatment based on techniques similar to cognitive/behavioral therapy methods. Unlike a structured program, therapy is not time-limited.

Individual cognitive/behavioral therapy requires that sufferers spend a substantial amount of time in the therapist's office dealing with the person's thoughts and feelings about the disorder. Many of these therapists also specialize in biofeedback, the process that helps sufferers learn to relax. This type of therapy also requires sufferers to spend a substantial amount of time and energy outside the office, working to face their fears.

Some therapists provide supported exposure; others suggest the outside use of a para-professional (usually recommended by them) or other support person (i.e., spouse, parent, friend, etc.) to help the sufferer face their fears.

This treatment method teaches anxiety management skills that will help sufferers in other aspects of their lives. There are a lot more anxiety disorder therapists than there are structured recovery treatment programs. Individual therapy allows the suffer to be treated alone rather than in a group setting. It also allows treatment to be started immediately rather than having the person wait weeks or months for a new group program to begin.

### *Family Therapy*

Basically, when family therapy is used to treat an anxiety disorder, it is not just family therapy per se but individual therapy focusing on the family situation. Thus this type of treatment is given by a therapist who is trained in both family therapy and anxiety disorder treatment that utilizes cognitive/behavioral anxiety reduction techniques. Again, treatment in not time-limited.

Family therapy is beneficial for those who have trouble

performing cognitive/behavioral treatment techniques because their family life is either chaotic or stressed by interpersonal conflicts.

### *Psychoanalytic Psychotherapy*

This type of therapy is useful when the sufferer has individual problems that need to be dealt with before the person can begin treating the anxiety disorder. The type of things that might need to be addressed might include a tendency to sabotage the person's own best endeavors, or the individual's habitual difficulty in completing tasks, or problems with commitment in general.

Psychoanalytic psychotherapy focuses on self-understanding. This therapy deals less with the sufferer's symptoms and more with the characteristics of the person's personality.

Psychoanalytic (insight) therapy is no guarantee that people will ever discover the origin of their anxiety disorder. Ironically the answer sometimes surfaces during or after their recovery from it. The main drawback of psychoanalytic psychotherapy is that it can last several years or longer. And although it helps sufferers with many areas of their lives by giving them insight into many things, it will not help them overcome their affliction.

### *Structured Treatment Program*

A structured treatment program is a time-limited comprehensive group course that teaches cognitive/behavioral therapy techniques to participants. Along with the workshop-oriented group meetings, this treatment includes exposure therapy either in a group setting (through field trips), individually with a support partner, or both. The treatment program is run by a psychiatrist, psychologist, therapist or a para-professional who is a recovered agoraphobic (when this is the case usually there is a health care professional on staff). Workshop sessions usually meet one to two hours, once a week, with the complete program lasting anywhere from eight to twenty-two weeks. Those who find a group setting and support among fellow sufferers beneficial may continue for additional follow-up group treatment.

The main goal is to help sufferers overcome their disorder by teaching them about their condition and what they can do about it. Sufferers spend some time during each session discussing their accomplishments and disappointments of the previous week. There are assignments between sessions, such as reading chapters in their workbook, practicing recovery techniques, doing exposure therapy (with a para-professional provided by the program or their own support person), and keeping a daily private diary, along with goal charts.

Some programs allow the sufferer's main support person—spouse, parent, adult child, or adult sibling—to attend the program with the sufferer. Of those who do, some provide both individuals separate time in their own support groups, along with the time spent together. Programs that include the spouse or other close relative have not only a higher recovery factor, but also a lower drop-out rate.

Sufferers recover faster in a group setting. It is also beneficial for sufferers (and their support people) to realize they are not alone in their disorder—others have the same problem. The value of the personal support and camaraderie among sufferers (and support people), along with the feedback that participants receive from one another, is beyond measure.

Many treatment programs offer home-study courses, combined with telephone help. While not affording the benefits of being in a group, excellent recovery results can still be obtained in many cases. Sufferers, however, sometimes have difficulty in maintaining motivation and staying on the program when they do not have a regular meeting to attend or someone to lead them.

## Choosing an Anxiety Disorder Therapist

*Who Can Be Therapists?*

Since agoraphobia and panic disorder can be treated by a variety of health care professionals, you are probably wondering what the differences are among mental health care professionals.

*Psychiatrists* are medical doctors who have several years of postgraduate training in the diagnosis and treatment of emotional and mental disorders. They treat a variety of problems ranging from mild emotional disorders to severe psychoses. The type of psychotherapy they practice ranges from short-term therapy to long-term psychoanalytic therapy. Psychiatrists can prescribe medication and hospitalize their patients. Some specialize in a particular field, such as child psychiatry.

*Psychologists* have an advanced degree in psychology. They deal with people's mental processes and behavior and are trained to perform psychological analysis and therapy along with research. They may perform psychotherapy with patients on an individual basis, as well as in groups. Some psychologists work in private practice, while others work as therapists for hospitals, mental-health centers, schools, even businesses. They usually have a doctorate, along with postdoctoral training, and their licensing requirements can vary depending on the state.

*Psychoanalysts* are usually medical doctors who have six to ten years of postgraduate training in psychoanalysis. American Psychoanalytic Association membership affords these professionals rigorous training in association-approved psychoanalytic institutes, but they can be trained by other institutes as well. Psychoanalysts who are M.D.s can prescribe medication, as well as hospitalize patients. However, experts say almost anybody can legally call themselves a psychoanalyst.

*Psychotherapists* usually help clients develop insight into their mental processes, teaching them to overcome maladaptive ways. These people can be trained, qualified, and licensed; however, they need not be. When choosing a psychotherapist, be sure to ask about background and training, checking with the proper local professional associations.

*Psychiatric Social Workers* may be in private practice or be the directors of clinics. Often they are actively involved with community programs dealing with drug abuse and such. They are the largest group of health care professionals in the health care field, and their licensing requirements vary from one state to another. Often, private treatment from social workers is not covered by health care insurance.

*Psychiatric Nurses* are R.N.s who hold advanced degrees. They may conduct individual therapy, as well as group therapy, in or out of a hospital setting.

*Para-Professionals* are trained to perform specific medical or teaching functions. They are not licensed to practice as professionals. Those who work in the anxiety disorder field are usually recovered agoraphobics. They may direct or teach a phobia program or assist a licensed medical professional who does. They may also do exposure therapy fieldwork with agoraphobia and anxiety disorder sufferers, usually under the supervision of a licensed medical professional.

No matter what type of therapist you and your loved one choose, you should both expect to receive the same courtesy and level of professionalism, including confidentiality, from all.

*Finding a Therapist*

Sufferers should pay attention to how well suited they are to the therapist, giving particular attention to their own feelings about this person. Sufferers should never hesitate to try several therapists before making a final decision.

To begin, call the therapist to get some general information. If you find the phone call isn't enough to get all your questions answered or to make a decision, request a consultation visit. Some therapists provide free consultations; others charge.

Here is a list of questions that Terrap recommends sufferers ask of a potential therapist. These can be asked either over the phone or in writing. If the answer to any of the first three questions is no, try another therapist; if yes, go on to the next question.

1. Do you treat people with agoraphobia, phobias, panic attack syndrome and obsessive-compulsive disorder?
2. Does the treatment involve cognitive/behavior therapy?
3. Is medication available from an experienced M.D.?
4. What training and experience have you and your staff had in treating these disorders?
5. Is treatment in groups available or is it individual therapy only? (Group is more effective and faster.)
6. Does treatment have a fixed length? If so, is advanced help

available afterwards? Is individual help available?

7. Is it possible to speak with a recovered client? (If the therapist has recovered clients, he can obtain permission for them to talk with a fellow sufferer.)

8. Do you include spouses in the treatment program? (If the spouse is included, the client is twice as likely to have a favorable and faster recovery.)

9. What does the therapy cost, and do you have any estimates as to what the average chances of a satisfactory recovery are? Also, if the course is dropped, how much of the cost is refundable?

10. Is treatment covered by insurance?

If you are satisfied with all the answers, ask for an individual session for diagnosis, evaluation, and personal feelings toward the therapist. (There may be a charge for evaluation, so ask.) Then ask the following questions of yourself and evaluate the therapist.

Rating Scale: 0 = strongly disagree  5 = strongly agree

| | | | | | | | |
|---|---|---|---|---|---|---|---|
| 1 | I feel comfortable with the therapist. | 0 | 1 | 2 | 3 | 4 | 5 |
| 2 | The therapist is easy to talk with. | 0 | 1 | 2 | 3 | 4 | 5 |
| 3 | The therapist answers my questions. | 0 | 1 | 2 | 3 | 4 | 5 |
| 4 | The therapist is willing to talk to other members of my family. | 0 | 1 | 2 | 3 | 4 | 5 |
| 5 | What the therapist says makes sense to me. | 0 | 1 | 2 | 3 | 4 | 5 |
| 6 | In general, my contact with the therapist gave me a more hopeful feeling. | 0 | 1 | 2 | 3 | 4 | 5 |
| 7 | The therapist has had anxiety attacks and has recovered. | 0 | 1 | 2 | 3 | 4 | 5 |

Total:_____

A total of 20 or below is unacceptable, 35 is excellent, and you can judge for yourself the acceptability of anything in between. Finding the right therapist is essential to recovery. Many therapists rely too much on medication and not enough on the psychological help. *Don't forget: Everyone has a right to a second opinion.*

Treatment is often expensive and can be a hardship when one has a limited income. For those who can't afford individual therapy or a group treatment program, there are clinics that offer a sliding pay scale, depending on the ability to pay. Government-sponsored clinics usually cost less. Also search for a university or hospital medical program that is conducting research in agoraphobia and panic disorder; research treatment is often free to study participants. However, before you enroll, make sure you fully understand the research program's conditions and techniques and find them agreeable.

Be wary of any therapist who advertises rates of cure, for example, therapists that claim to cure 90 to 100 percent of their clients. While it's true that agoraphobia is a highly treatable condition and 90 percent of sufferers can overcome the disorder, no one can guarantee how an individual will do in therapy.

## What to Look for in a Recovery Treatment Program

There are certain things a good recovery treatment program should contain. According to Dr. Hardy, the best recovery programs will provide the following:

1. Evaluation, diagnosis, and prognosis of the condition, along with the time treatment requires.

2. Education about the disorder, why the client has it, what to do about it, and what not to do about it.

3. Behavior therapy that includes relaxation, desensitization, and especially in-vivo exposure.

4. Availability of medication and closely monitored usage to prevent addiction.

5. Cognitive therapy to help clients change erroneous thinking patterns such as negative thinking and self-defeating attitudes.

6. Therapy in groups of other agoraphobic/panic disorder victims, along with support groups.

7. Education of the spouse and inclusion of the spouse in therapy with the agoraphobic person.

8. Individual help available, as well as telephone help and advanced help.

9. Field instructor availability.

Some additional items a program should contain are: instruction on coping skills to help clients learn how to cope with their new type of life; negotiation skills to help clients learn to discuss their views with others, the end goal being to come to a mutual agreement about issues important to meeting their recovery needs; instruction in communication skills to help clients better explain themselves to others who either don't understand or need to understand their problem; and the teaching of goal setting skills to help clients learn how to set and keep recovery goals.

### How to Know if the Treatment Is Working

According to the Anxiety Disorder Association of America, "As a general rule you should see some improvement within twelve to sixteen weeks. If you are not making substantial progress after three or four months of treatment you should talk with your therapist and determine if you need to change the treatment plan." It may be time to find a new therapist if sufferers find talking with their therapist about slow progress only leads to an unsatisfactory conclusion, or if sufferers find they are repeatedly going over the same material with no progress in sight.

You'll know the chosen treatment plan is working if (1) there is continual improvement, even though at times it may seem snail-like, (2) the sufferer has not lost track of his or her recovery goal, and (3) the sufferer continues to maintain a therapeutic alliance with the therapist. Although the time recovery takes largely depends on the individual and his or her circumstances, when these three elements are present the length of time the treatment plan lasts is of minimal importance.

One important note: In the beginning sufferers don't often notice their own improvement, because it is small. Therefore they must depend on the feedback from others (if they are in a group) or their support people to help them recognize the signs of progress.

## TIPS FOR A SUCCESSFUL PROGRAM

Enrollment in a recovery program or obtaining an anxiety

disorder therapist doesn't guarantee sufferers a successful recovery. What does is the person's strong determination to get well. Sufferers only get out of treatment what they put into it. They must use and practice the recovery techniques outlined in their chosen plan of treatment in order to develop the skills that will reduce their anxiety. Following is a list of recovery tips that will help make the sufferer's treatment of choice a success.

· Be willing to put forth the effort it takes to recover. Work hard at learning new skills. Don't wait for someone else to fix the problem. Make recovery one's first priority. Schedule time so that recovery comes first before anything else.

· Make a commitment to follow all the instructions laid out by the treatment program or therapist. Commitment to the chosen treatment plan is crucial to recovery. If you procrastinate, discuss this tendency with the therapist.

· Be patient with the recovery program, the therapist, one's support person and most of all oneself. Recovery takes time; progress comes in small stages.

· Listen to the therapist or program director, along with the feedback of others in the group. Fellow sufferers often seem to have the ability see and understand the sufferer's mental attitudes and behavior better than this person does.

· Read and reread all the materials on the disorder. All programs have a suggested reading list. Learn all you can about the disorder and how to overcome it. Recovery depends on how well sufferers understand their own condition.

· Give the therapist or program a chance. Certain legitimate recovery techniques may seem unusual, but they work. Do the best you can to follow all directions. Don't try to improvise or make alterations unless the therapist recommends it.

· Be willing to make necessary lifestyle changes. "One of the reasons people don't recover," Dr. Hardy said, "is their failure to make changes."

· Communicate progress or lack of it to the group and the therapist. It helps to get a pat on the back for what's been accomplished—praise and encouragement are great incentives. Realize that lack of progress provides a learning opportunity.

· Participate actively in the recovery process and ask questions.

· Keep that therapeutic alliance with the therapist or group leader alive. It's important for both the therapist and the patient to know what each expects from one another during treatment and to carry on a collaborative effort. Mingle with group members. Don't be a loner. Fellow sufferers provide excellent support.

· Use positive affirmations daily to help overcome negative thinking that can interfere with recovery. Along with this, the most effective way to change negative thinking and behavior is to associate with those who have more positive patterns of thinking.

· Reduce anxiety through daily relaxation exercises. Be willing to face fears and risk uncomfortable bodily sensations from time to time.

· Practice, practice, practice. Continually practice the recovery skills being learned. Dr. Hardy said, "Recovery is like a skill: if you use it, it will improve; if not, it will become rusty." And do all the homework. It's there for a good reason.

· Give yourself permission to make mistakes and use them as an opportunity to learn. Plus, don't compare your recovery with those of others in the group. Everybody recovers at their own speed.

· Refrain from making excuses for not performing the recovery techniques. If you continually makes excuses, ask yourself why. Are you afraid to recover? Are there secondary gains to keeping the disorder? Excuses only prolong recovery.

· Refrain from being your own therapist. Anxiety disorder therapists are equipped to make the proper diagnoses and to prescribe the right help. In addition, be as honest as possible with the therapist and with yourself. Honestly accepting your anxiety disorder helps to change it. Be honest about your own performance. Are you conscientious about attending therapy or group sessions regularly, reading the program materials, doing the homework, and practicing the recovery techniques? Or could you be doing a better job? Are you open to new ideas, or have you remained too rigid in your thinking? These issues play an important part in how much one improves during treatment.

Recovery requires a lot of courage on the sufferer's part.

Facing fears is very scary, so don't be disappointed if these suggestions aren't always followed. Expect some reluctance now and then. As a support person, you cannot make the sufferer do any of these things. What you can do, however, is try your best to help the person to accomplish them.

## CHAPTER FIVE

# How Agoraphobia Affects the Family

*"Virtually all human change begins with attitude."*

—*Dr. Wayne W. Dyer, Pulling Your Own Strings*

No family member is ever left untouched by agoraphobia and panic disorder. Those affected say it is just as hard for them to live with the problem as it is for the sufferer.

Agoraphobia affects the whole family. Often there is one reaction from the spouse, another from the children, and still another from relatives and friends—which I will consider in this book to be a larger extended family, and sometimes part of the family support team.

## INITIAL FAMILY REACTIONS

Through many years of treating men and women who suffer from agoraphobia and panic disorder, Dr. Hardy found that the victim's family (and sometimes friends) nearly always go through a sequence of events when agoraphobia and/or panic disorder first strikes. Within this sequence there are seven stages, not all of which occur in each instance.

1. *Disbelief.* When agoraphobia first strikes, the husband, wife, or other family member is absolutely shocked. He or she can't understand why the sufferer can't do the simple things the sufferer was able to perform only a short time before. For example, when one husband found out about his wife's condition, he told me, "At the time, I thought it was B.S." This may sound harsh, but it is a good example of how some family members feel.

After the initial shock wears off and the spouse or other member accepts the fact that the sufferer can't help being afflicted, he or she usually tries to be helpful. However, the problem is that this individual often doesn't understand the nature of phobias. As a result, he or she tries to use logic and objective reasoning on an emotional problem.

One husband said, "I couldn't understand why my wife couldn't talk herself out of the problem since she talked herself into it in the first place." In applying logical thinking, he told his wife that there was no reason for her to be afraid of driving a car, going over a bridge, waiting in line in a grocery store, or going to a movie theater. He also told her to pull herself together and grow up.

Of course, the sufferer understands the logic, but his or her deep-down panic always seems to prevail. For this reason, well-meaning suggestions aren't helpful. In fact, they may well be detrimental. Any time a family member uses a "logical" approach, the sufferer begins to feel put down and criticized. As a result, the anxiety level increases and the disorder gets worse.

For example, when panic attacks became a regular event in my own life, I began to ask, "What's wrong with me?" I remember standing in the middle of a large shopping mall, surrounded by stores I once loved to visit, yet all I wanted to do was run for the nearest exit.

It certainly didn't help when my husband tried to calm me down. His reason didn't diminish my growing fear of the places where my panic attacks occurred. My world deteriorated around me. Life became a struggle. And with each passing day I became more afraid. I also became extremely depressed. All of this was very frustrating for my husband. He and other members of my family tried to help, but they didn't know how.

When everything relatives have tried doesn't work, confusion sets in.

2. *Frustration.* Often the family member can't help, because object reasoning and logic don't work. It seems to this person that the sufferer isn't trying hard enough to get better. Sometimes this causes the family member to become angry, because his or her efforts don't produce results. Desperate, he or she demands more effort on the part of the sufferer. This demand belittles the agoraphobic further and intensifies the problem. As a result, the well-meaning relative eventually gives up and starts thinking about finding another solution.

For example, George, whose wife was agoraphobic, expressed concern about his anger and asked how to deal with it. "I found myself in a real dilemma," he told me. "I can suffer in silence, or I can state my feelings and needs. Either way, it's a no-win situation." Another spouse added, "If I say that my wife's disorder is sometimes not very comfortable for me to be around, she feels I'm being critical." Both men felt that if they disclosed their feelings, even in a kind way, it complicated the entire problem.

When the family member gives up and starts thinking about another way to solve the problem, his or her reactions will have one of the following results.

3. *Failure.* Because the family member has no idea what to do, he or she often experiences a feeling of failure and frequently wants to stop trying to help. This adds to the sufferer's feelings of insecurity and often intensifies the agoraphobia or panic disorder.

At this point this individual often assumes the attitude of "It's your problem, so do it yourself and let me alone" or "I can't handle this—count me out."

When I was in the Terrap program, I met a fellow agoraphobic whose husband had this attitude. At the beginning he attended meetings with her. Soon he came only every other week, then finally not at all. "He considers my condition an inconvenience," she told me. "He hears but doesn't listen. He doesn't want to understand or help." Time and again he would put her in situations with which he knew she was uncomfortable, then verbally attack her for the inconvenience she caused him.

Attitudes can change. The husband mentioned eariler who thought his wife's condition was B.S. believed the disorder was her problem. Later, when he became more involved in her recovery, he resolved to help.

4. *Emotional Separation.* When the family member is a husband or wife, he or she may remain with the sufferer but create a separate existence. This spouse may become preoccupied with business or other activities. Some husbands or wives may even start taking separate vacations. While at home, such persons often feel remorse for pulling away from the ill spouse when they are needed most. So rather than spend time at home, the non-suffering individual avoids it. The separation between the two increases, causing both to feel guilt and depression. Since the sufferer already feels unwanted, inadequate, and in danger of being rejected, this exaggerates the problem.

For instance, when Cindy's family first found out about her agoraphobia, they felt sorry for her and stayed home because she was afraid to be alone. As time passed the family became restless. Annoyed with the problem, they began to leave her completely alone. "I was crying out for help," she said, "but they were tired of dealing with the same old problem."

To make matters worse, her husband decided that her disorder was just a play for sympathy.

However, no one develops this disorder to get attention, to be taken care of, or as a way of relating to others. As Dr. Hardy said, "Secondary gains can occur later and become a way of relating, depending on the response from people closely associated, but in the beginning it is motivated by survival, fears, and discomfort avoidance."

In many cases, the spouse becomes upset because of the guilt and depression he or she is feeling, in part wondering if he or she might have caused the disorder. Becoming angry, this person verbally attacks not only the ailing spouse but sometimes the children. Consequently, this person no longer lives up to his or her own expectations of marriage and parenthood. This deepens his or her depression. At this point such an individual needs help as much as the ailing spouse does.

5. *Divorce or Coexistence.* With married couples, if the separation continues, the marriage will be threatened and often end in divorce (this also applies to cases where the extended family essentially breaks apart). Surprisingly, however, Dr. Hardy found that while there are divorces caused by agoraphobia, there seem to be fewer divorces among this group than among the general public.

For some sufferers, divorce is a step toward recovery, because it puts them on their own. Once he or she realizes there is no help, that individual begins to help him- or herself get better.

In one case, Pat and her husband, who had been married many years, were getting a divorce as a direct result of her agoraphobia and panic disorder. "Since we used to go so many places together," she said, "Joe simply couldn't handle staying home and started going without me. After about a year of this he found another woman." Although at first it seemed to be the end of the world with Joe no longer around, Pat became more determined to recover and sought help for the disorder. Within a short time she started to get better.

It is not uncommon for someone to love an agoraphobic partner but still leave this person because of the affliction. Agoraphobia can interfere with a couple's activities to such an extent that it wrecks the relationship. The love is still there, but the restrictions put too much strain on the marriage (and sometimes on extended family relationships). However, if the sufferer improves and starts expanding his or her world, this often improves the family relationship.

Some couples choose just to separate emotionally. Adjusting their lives to this separation, they continue living together in a peaceful coexistence. Sadly, it is an unsatisfactory system for both people.

6. *Caretaker.* Sometimes, the husband or wife (or other family member) may decide to continue the marriage (or relationship) and become the sufferer's caretaker. Although this arrangement happens primarily between husband and wife, it can also happen between the sufferer and any other family member or friend.

The spouse or family member adopts the attitude "I love him/her, so I will adjust to the problem." As caretaker, the family member does everything for the sufferer. The agoraphobic no longer needs to face his or her fears or deal with the disorder. If the sufferer has been in therapy he or she often withdraws. The family member does all the shopping, all the driving, all the entertaining, or stays home, sometimes literally enslaving him- or herself to the sufferer.

The caretaker wants to be available whenever possible. As a result this person gives up doing things he or she enjoys. For instance, a husband or other male relative may no longer bowl, go hunting or fishing, or play golf. A wife or female relative who assumes a caretaker role may also give up her outside activities. If, in a panic, the sufferer phones the caretaker relative at work, he or she rushes right home. This family member often becomes resentful, because it is impossible to do everything, and nothing gets done satisfactorily.

If the family member is a husband or wife, the couple's social life begins to suffer. They stop planning fun activities with friends. As one husband said, "My wife didn't want me to tell friends about her disorder. I felt I was caught in the middle. I get tired of making excuses, but what do you do?"

Eventually, the sufferer and the caretaker become totally isolated from others. In lieu of sharing experiences that once strengthened the relationship, they now share anxiety.

Since the caretaker has created a comfortable *phobic nest*, this intensifies the problem. Although he or she tries to fill every need and request, the demands keep growing. Any recovery stops, and in most cases the disorder regresses. This is a bad case of over-love by a family member.

Actually, the phobic nest is an excellent way for the sufferer to obtain security. It is important for the beginning of recovery. But I can tell you from experience that recovery does not take place within this nest, only away from it. (I will deal thoroughly with the phobic nest in Chapter 6.)

7. *"Our Problem."* Sharing the problem is the most desirable attitude. All the family members decide to make the problem "our problem" and work it out together. This attitude of "Let's make the problem our problem, not just the sufferer's problem" strengthens the family relationship. The agoraphobia and panic disorder is then worked out without pressure, demands, rejection, or threats. The family team learns to understand the sufferer's problem, discovers the causes, and decides what to do to help. This provides the best

environment for recovery.

Even though a panic attack is not the support person's fault, it is still a joint problem. One mother whose married daughter was afflicted with agoraphobia said, "My being there made her feel a little more secure. We learned about the problem together and worked on it side by side. This brought us closer as a family. It also helped me discover that she wasn't nuts."

Making my problem "our problem" in a family-supported program was one of the main reasons my recovery was so successful. Ed, my husband, was always there when I needed him. I knew he could be trusted as my support person. This gave me a world of confidence when entering fearful situations. He was there through the good days as well as bad. He filled my anxious world with positive words of encouragement, rather than negative criticism. Not only did his love and support help me recover, but as we worked together to overcome my problem our relationship strengthened.

## THE SPECIAL PROBLEMS OF CHILDREN

Children in the family pose a special problem. Do you tell them or not? If so, when and how do you explain, and how will they react? Also, what can you do to help them deal with the problem?

When panic attacks and agoraphobia hit a family, the first reaction is to hide the problem from the children. I must admit that I reacted in this way. I believed that it was in the children's best interest (and mine) to keep the affliction hidden. My son Tim, who was eleven years old, was quiet, shy, and over-protected. I worried constantly that if he discovered the truth he would come down with the disorder. I also didn't want Tom, nineteen, and Gary, twenty, to think their mother was less than the perfectly normal mom they remembered when they lived at home.

When I was in the Terrap program, Dr. Leman told me not to worry. As I started to recover and change my behavior, Tim would see this, and modeling from my example, would open up and become more outgoing. I didn't really believe him. Although I made a few attempts at revealing the problem, I ended up keeping the disorder to myself.

The problem was easy to hide from Gary and Tom, but Tim, who lived at home, watched as I went through the downhill process of change. He didn't understand why. During this time, he began to become more and more like me. However, because of the Terrap program I attended once a week, he learned about my problem gradually. He watched me getting worse, but he also saw me turn around and begin to get better and better. At this point, I was able to tell him about my disorder and discovered he understood completely. As I became better, Tim did exactly what Dr. Leman said he would do: model after me. He followed my lead. He soon became happy and normal, not the same scared little boy he had been.

The older boys were a different problem. They weren't around twenty-four hours a day, but they certainly put different demands on me. My oldest son, Gary, wanted me to help him pick out a ski outfit as a birthday present for his girlfriend Stephanie. I was sure he would never understand if I had a panic attack and had to rush home. I had feigned being sick twice, and he was getting tired of my excuses. Finally my husband Ed suggested that he drive us, and if something happened he would say I was sick and take me home. That problem was easy to solve.

However, as Gary and Stephanie's relationship became more serious, they wanted my husband and me to meet her parents. I got through a terrible night with her parents at a special Italian restaurant where the romance began. Every bite of food stuck in my throat, but nobody knew I was having trouble.

The Tupperware party Stephanie chose to give, however, was a disaster. I was becoming more and more housebound at this point. When Stephanie's mother, Jo Allyn, came by to pick me up for the party, panic struck, and my husband had to tell her I became suddenly ill with a stomach flu attack. That evening I cried myself to sleep.

Gary became more and more irritated, because I kept making excuses as to why we couldn't get together with Stephanie and her parents. The situation did change, albeit slowly.

One day as I started to get better, Gary dropped by and began to tell me about seeing a television show about panic attacks and how they affected people's lives. Before I knew it, I had told him my problem. His first reaction was: How do you know? Then, are you sure? Why hadn't he known? Could he get it? There were many questions. After that, I was able to tell Tom. As it turned out, both had already sensed something was wrong and had discussed it.

Looking back, I realize I shouldn't have hidden the disorder. I could have saved myself much stress and anxiety. When they finally knew, my boys still considered me to be good old mom, and they still loved me just as much.

## Can Children Catch the Disorder?

The agoraphobic often avoids telling his or her children, because he or she feels that they might contract it. Is there any truth to this? In his book *Overcoming Agoraphobia,* Dr. Alan Goldstein says that daughters in particular are at risk of developing panic attacks when they grow up in a home with a parent who has those symptoms. Dr. Barlow also reports that mothers who display fears of airplanes, thunderstorms, and such often have kids with similar fears. "The seeds of fear," he said, "only grow when they fall on fertile soil."

Dr. Hardy believed children can inherit the timidity that makes them vulnerable. Following general genetic rules, he said that if only one parent has agoraphobia, usually only one out of four children will also have it, usually a child of the same sex as the phobic parent. He felt that if both parents have agoraphobia, all of their children would have the problem to some degree.

Attempts by agoraphobic parents to hide the disorder are never a complete protection. The children still pick up the avoidance. Experts say if parents find children suffering from any intense or prolonged fears or missing out on important aspects of life because of phobic avoidance, the child's situation has become serious and warrants intervention.

Although research is still ongoing, evidence seems to indicate that at least some of the problem is inherited. Experts don't really know, however, whether the condition is inherited genetically or comes from environmental influences. I'm inclined to believe the disorder stems from both.

## What's the Reaction to Not Being Told?

Even though children of parents who suffer from agoraphobia and panic disorder often sense something is wrong, they aren't sure exactly what. Unfortunately, many sufferers are often ashamed of having the ailment and aren't sure what their children might think of them if they knew. In addition, some are afraid that if they tell the kids, neighbors or other people will find out.

The real question is How do children react to being in an agoraphobic family? This question was the object of a study by Judy Brooks, who headed a program for children of agoraphobics supervised by the Knopf Company in Plymouth, Michigan. The study group consisted of eight girls and boys ranging from about five to eleven years of age. Here are some of the things she discovered.

When the agoraphobic parent doesn't go to events most other parents go to, such as soccer and baseball, the child often feels he or she is not worthy of the parent's love. Soon that youngster begins to feel that he or she deserves to be treated this way. In addition, if the parents aren't there when children think they should be, the children often feel it's because they did something wrong. They wonder why their moms or dads aren't like other parents.

These children also often suffer from low self-esteem. Because of the disorder, the focus is on the person who is ill. Consequently the children don't receive the parental attention they would receive in a healthier family. When this happens, these children begin to believe their needs are not as important as the needs of the adults in the house.

Besides this problem, children of agoraphobic parents used illness as a defense more often than other children. They complained of having a headache or other ailments. This made sense in terms of agoraphobia: The family system says it's alright to be sick and it is an accepted behavior to cancel events because of sickness.

In the study groups, when the child didn't want to discuss something the group was discussing, that child would often become "sick." In addition, the study group itself had to be canceled for one week because too many kids were "sick." Children of dysfunctional families, just as those from alcoholic homes, are often tough and don't want anyone to think anyone is wrong with them, but Brooks found these children didn't do that.

Most of the children in the study had little access to their own feelings and couldn't express them. However, when Brooks started to talk about how they felt, what was going on at home, and what they could do to make things better, the kids lit up like light bulbs.

Some of these children could also talk at great length about what their parents would and would not do and why. This helped the children who didn't understand their parent's disorder and didn't know why mom went to phobia group meetings or why dad got angry at mom for not going places where he wanted to go. In practice, however, Dr. Hardy discovered that when the agoraphobic gets stronger and recovers, the child usually returns to normal.

## To Tell or Not to Tell?

Most of the time parents think their children will survive despite everything, even if the problem is kept from them. Most kids do, but it's much healthier if the parents share the problem with them. Children are perceptive. Most know when their parents are feeling good or bad. Unfortunately, parents don't often give their children credit for what they know. If, by talking to their children, parents help them validate their feelings and sort them out for them, children are much less vulnerable.

Explains Jerilyn Ross, President of the Anxiety Disorder Association of America, "Children are better off knowing. Many people with phobias try to protect their children. As a result, the kids never learn it's OK to be frightened. Children need to know adults feel scared, too. They need to know it's important to express their feelings. Unfortunately, if parents are overcautious with children because of their own fears, the children may soon pick up this fearfulness."

## How Do You Explain It?

The kinds of questions children need answered about agoraphobia and panic disorder are different from the kind adults need answered. Children do not need technical explanations; they do, however, need to know why their parent didn't go to the baseball game, or why dad was yelling at mom because she wouldn't go to church, or why mom always stays home. Here are some ways to approach the problem:

Some experts believe you should explain it to young children in terms of scary things children can relate to: the bogey man, being afraid of the dark, or strange noises. Tell them that grown-ups too can be afraid of things they don't really have to be afraid of. Point out the fact that what may be frightening to one person might not scare another at all. This often helps children understand the parent's fears and feel better about their own.

You can also talk to children about agoraphobia and panic disorder, as Ms. Brooks did, in terms of other diseases that children know about: chicken pox, measles, flu. Point out their symptoms: some last a long time, others go away; some come from a virus, some from something you ate. Then point out that agoraphobia is similar to this, but it is a disorder, not a disease. Finally ask questions such as: Did anybody blame you when you had chicken pox or flu? Let the child answer. Then point out that this disease was out of their control, and so is yours. Brooks found that while young children easily accept this explanation, older children don't as easily as they often get angry at the parent's disorder.

When talking to children, explain the problem to them just the way it is. For instance, you might say, "Have you ever noticed when I do this and this? Do you have any idea why? I haven't been able to tell you before, because I get so frightened. Even though I don't think there is any real danger, I feel it, so I go by my feelings." While all of these methods are helpful, in practice, you must tailor your approach to the individual child.

## If You Decide Not to Tell

What if you decide not to tell the children at all? Many experts feel this may be alright under some circumstances. Dr. Manual D. Zane, founder and director of the Phobia Clinic in White Plains, New York, believes that truth and reality are the most helpful approach, but children shouldn't be told unless the parents themselves feel they can handle it. "It depends on the factors involved within the phobic's life."

Moreover, other family members shouldn't tell children about the disorder unless the afflicted parent feels comfortable with them doing so. If telling the children adds too much stress to a sufferer's already stressful condition, then the time isn't right.

This was true in my case. My youngest son, Tim, would have been better off knowing at the outset, but I personally couldn't have handled it, nor did I want my husband to tell anyone.

A few sufferers choose never to tell the children. A Pennsylvania woman who suffered from agoraphobia and panic attacks for almost forty years said that her children still don't know. "I never told because I believed in suggestibility and thought I might transfer it to them." Apparently her children suffered no ill effects.

### Can Children Help?

Dr. Hardy found that it helps children to be allowed to take part in the recovery process. This often makes them more accepting and tolerant. They should be allowed to help set goals, participate in reality testing, and assist the sufferer in other positive ways. I would, however, beware of role reversal, whereby the child ends up taking care of the parent.

Since the parent is, in effect, modeling for the child (how to recover from the disorder rather than how to avoid it), Dr. Hardy believed it will help keep the child from becoming phobic. In my case, my son Tim overcame his fears by watching me overcome mine. It depends on the individual child and should be a judgment call on the part of the parent.

Because kids often feel that they caused the problem or could have prevented it, they need to understand they are not to blame. Make sure they know no one is mad at them and they had nothing to do with causing the problem. Let them know too that sometimes it's alright to be angry at how the disorder makes the afflicted parent act.

Give children permission to talk about the disorder and what's going on in the family, so if they aren't getting enough attention, they at least know why. This improves communication, helps eliminate any guilt children feel, and builds their self-esteem.

In addition, if the parents can't give the child the attention he or she needs, then the team needs to do it or arrange for the child to get attention elsewhere. A grandmother or aunt, for instance, can drive them where they need to go or arrange for someone else to do it, perhaps with the mother or father of the children's friends. With a little attention and sensitivity on the part of parents, children will come through this crisis much better than most parents think they will.

## WHAT ABOUT EXTENDED FAMILY AND CLOSE FRIENDS?

Those who suffer often avoid relatives (outside of the husband/wife, mother/father structure) and drift away from friends. When they hide their condition, these friends and relatives often think the sufferer is being unfriendly or just likes staying home. Eventually others stop coming around or, tired of being turned down, stop asking. The sufferer's and the spouse's social life becomes virtually nonexistent. This leads to more isolation and loneliness for both. This also deprives the sufferer of what he or she needs most: moral support and understanding from others.

Sometimes when the sufferer keeps his or her condition secret, it not only makes their lives more difficult but can stand in the way of overcoming the disorder.

I kept my disorder hidden from others for a long time. My husband Ed respected my wish for secrecy and kept my secret within the family.

Stephanie, my son's girlfriend, was the first outsider I told. One morning, she called and invited me to go with her to a local farmer's market, formerly one of my favorite places. Feeling brave, I agreed.

By the time Stephanie arrived, I had become extremely anxious. When she greeted me with a big hug, I suddenly told her about my disorder. "If you get panicky and can't stay," she told me, "we'll leave." Her compassion gave me the confidence to try.

## Chapter 5

When Stephanie parked the car in the parking lot, my anxiety rose. But with her at my side, I felt I could handle it. The further we got from the car, the more nervous I became.

As she picked out baskets at one stand, panic suddenly overwhelmed me. My stomach began to cramp; I knew diarrhea would follow. I rushed off, saying, "Steph, I need to use the restroom." When she found me, I told her I had to leave. "No problem," she said as she put her arms around me. From that day on I had another confidant and support person. The network was growing.

I continued to go places with her. Sometimes I was successful and sometimes I failed, but she never made fun of my peculiar behavior or became angry and complained when I had to return home. Her positive reaction led me to tell others.

Keeping anxiety and fears locked up exaggerates them and makes them more terrifying. When a sufferer discloses his or her fears to others, he or she will become more objective. This helps bring the fears under control.

In my interviews I found that many sufferers had experiences similar to mine. One of the people I talked to, Louise from Kentucky, said, "It was hard telling others about my disorder, but it was even harder having to lie." Missie from California said, "Telling friends is a risk. Inevitably some will distance themselves from you. But I don't regret telling those who ran away, because the more people I told, the stronger and less anxious I became."

As Hilde from California found, there are added benefits in telling others. "Besides my parents, my close friends know and are supportive when I talk about my ups and downs. They cheer me on. There is no way to explain that special feeling. If I had kept quiet, my feelings about my successes during recovery would be different. People wouldn't know how much each success—driving the car, going to the store—meant to me."

Lydia from Illinois said, "The worst thing that happened was that some people ignored my discussing agoraphobia because they could not relate to it. They preferred to talk about themselves."

Betty, another Californian, said, "Those closest to me felt they might have contributed to the condition. So they ignored it." Joan from Pennsylvania wished she had told only her husband and children, for her mother and other relatives ridiculed all her attempts at recovery.

Nora, a West Virginia resident, was very open and honest and told everyone about her ailment, but no one understood. "Except for my closest relatives and a few friends, most didn't want to help. Eventually they just eliminated me from their social plans altogether."

Those relatives or friends who try to keep the sufferer's problem hidden from others find it difficult. Here are a few comments: Barbara, a support person to a male friend, found keeping the disorder hidden very difficult. "I got tired of making excuses and lying to cover up his problem, so I told his sister. I also told several close friends and my mother. I don't feel it's my responsibility to cover up for him."

Jim, whose wife Jane suffered from agoraphobia, said, "Telling family was not difficult, but because they denied the problem, didn't accept the treatment method, and thought she should recover faster than she did, it became a sore point. In addition, because she chose to tell certain friends and not others, it was hard to explain why we often didn't show up where we had promised we would or why we didn't go in the first place. This caused me anxiety."

Some people will not understand the problem and will respond in a negative or discouraging way. But the reaction you get from people can be totally unexpected. The friends you least envision being supportive may be the ones who stand by, while others you thought you could depend upon most may turn away.

Those who are afflicted, however, do themselves a disservice by hiding the disorder from good friends. The more support a sufferer has, the larger the recovery network and the easier it is to overcome the disorder. It is important to begin to tell people about the problem. This untraps the sufferer and allows him or her to try new situations.

## Explaining the Disorder

Sometimes it seems to matter less *who* you tell than *how* you tell them. Sufferers who understand and accept their fears as a treatable stress-related problem are the ones who get the most acceptance. Those who believe that something is fundamentally wrong with them and feel ashamed often tell others in a self-destructive way, resulting in a negative response.

For most people, a brief explanation is best. However, when recruiting other relatives or friends as support team members, try to be as clear as possible when explaining what the condition is and how it is treated.

Explain with an example: Many people fail to understand the fears of agoraphobia, so outline it in terms they can understand. Jerilyn Ross, for instance, says that most people understand the fear you might have standing in the middle of the highway with cars coming at you at a hundred miles an hour. So explain it in those terms. Then explain that sometimes when you are standing talking to a friend or driving along the freeway, you suddenly have those same feelings for no reason—that's how a phobic person feels. Sometimes this occurs by just thinking about the situation.

Another example I have used is, "When driving, have you ever almost been hit by another car?" Many people have and usually say yes. Then I say, "You know the anxious feelings that rush through your body at that particular moment, the rush of adrenaline? Well that's what a panic attack feels like, except it comes on unexpectedly, without cause."

After my listener understands, I explain that people who experience panic attacks usually start avoiding the places where they have occurred. Eventually, the world grows smaller and smaller. I use claustrophobia as a comparison, but I explain that unlike fearing one thing, agoraphobics fear a variety of places and circumstances. Most people seem to understand this.

For those who have a difficult time telling others, Terrap recommends using a "Dear Person" letter. This letter briefly explains that the sender has agoraphobia, what agoraphobia is, and that the sufferer is under treatment. It details the needs of the sufferer, then asks for that individual's help. See Figure 5 for a sample letter. Many sufferers find a letter useful, because they don't have to retell the problem personally or face the shock of others.

If you are a member of the support team rather than the

## Figure 5

Dear _____,

I want to tell you something about myself. I have a problem with a  type of anxiety called agoraphobia. This is not a mental illness but a kind of anxiety that causes panic attacks.

Although one in twenty-five people suffer from agoraphobia, few people have heard of the condition. It is difficult for me to talk about, but sharing this information with you is important to me.

Agoraphobia is similar to claustrophobia, except that panic attacks can be triggered by many things: crowds, distance from home, freeways, bridges, and many other situations. I can neither anticipate nor control these anxiety attacks. Because these attacks are extremely uncomfortable, sometimes terrifying, and always embarrassing, I have been avoiding situations that might arouse them.

I have found help for this problem and am making progress. At this point I am able to do some things and want to do even more, but I still need a way out of situations that are frightening to me. I have found that when other people understand that I may need to leave an uncomfortable situation, I can do better and it helps my recovery.

It is extremely important to me to feel free to leave any given situation at any time, no matter how innocuous the situation may appear. I don't ask that you understand my condition, but I would appreciate your help.

In telling you this I am not soliciting your sympathy, but I would like your moral support as I work toward recovery. I realize that the way I confront the problem may seem confusing and even inappropriate to you. Be assured that I have been treated by other methods but have found that the system I am now using is helping me to recover. By your acceptance you will be working with me in overcoming this problem.

Sincerely,

sufferer, you need to use caution when advising the agoraphobic about whom to tell and when. Above all, don't try to push your afflicted loved one into revealing his or her disorder. Victims must do what they feel is best. Often the sufferer needs time to build up self-confidence. As the sufferer learns more about the disorder and starts to work at overcoming it, explaining the problem to others will become easier.

# The Basics of Good Support

*The most effective weapon you have for wiping out
fear and anxiety is your own determination.*

## UNDERSTANDING THE FUNDAMENTALS
## OF SUPPORT

In the family-supported recovery plan, every family member
plays a part in the recovery process. As a team, you utilize your
strengths by working together on the suffer's problem. The solution
to this problem then becomes the family team's number-one goal.

The participants in a family support team include one main support person—often the spouse—and several alternate or side supporters, such as children, brothers, sisters, parents, and other relatives
or close friends. The main support person is the lead man or woman.

Attitude is everything in treating agoraphobia. When the family
team members understand the importance of attitude and the need to
support the sufferer with a positive one throughout the recovery period, the recovery time is shortened significantly. On the other hand,
the wrong attitude and treatment on the part of the family team can
not only stop recovery in its tracks, but can also reverse any progress the sufferer may have made.

After attitude, the primary job of support people is to help the agoraphobic progressively face his or her fears so they eventually disappear. You will often be required to be with the sufferer when he or she confronts the situations that induce panic. You are there to reassure your loved one, to help maintain a sense of security, and to encourage and motivate him or her. You are also there to help the sufferer label the fear  on a scale of 0 to 10 and to remind him or her of the behavioral skills he or she is learning—whether it be from a book like this one, a self-help group, or a recovery program.

To be a good support person you do not need to hold advanced degrees or be an expert in psychology. What you do need is interest, patience, understanding, and a willingness to help the sufferer to help him- or herself. You are not expected to—nor should you—try to be a therapist to your partner. However, it is important for you to fully understand and be familiar with the recovery process. It's also important for you to be careful only to offer the time and support you are willing to give, because to help the suffer, once you begin, you must consistently follow through.

Sometimes it's not an easy job to be a support person, especially if you are the main one. At times it can be frustrating and demanding. Your role and all that it requires may even begin to make you feel uncertain about the job. This is only natural. Being a support person is very hard but very rewarding.

Understand that your close emotional ties to the sufferer will give you and other members of the family support team influence over this person's feelings and behavior. This can affect your role as a support person. Sometimes your close attachment can make you too emotionally involved. You may empathize too much with the sufferer when he or she experiences phobic distress. Thus, you may give in too soon when he or she hesitates while confronting a phobic situation, or when he or she wants to miss a practice session because it is more comfortable to stay at home. You might even let this person back away from a problem rather than work at solving it, because it's too painful.

On the other hand, your close attachment can lead you to take the opposite approach and be so enthusiastic and eager for your loved one's next recovery step that you unknowingly push this person into taking the step before he or she is ready, thereby forcing the sufferer beyond the pace he or she is comfortable with.

Nonetheless, your closeness to the sufferer is what enables you to be more aware than a professional would be of any special areas of difficulty this person will have when facing his or her fears. Consequently, as long as you follow the basics of good support, you can be of more benefit to the sufferer during practice sessions than any professional ever could.

It is important to know that it can take several months or even longer before you begin to see significant progress. Recovery is a one-step-at-a-time process, and the sufferer must go only at a pace he or she is comfortable with. Some sufferers take longer to recover than others, for each situation is different. At a minimum, the lead support person needs to work with and help the sufferer at least three times a week, spending several hours with this person each time as he or she works at confronting fears. Other members of the family support team need to be available to fill in for, or alternate with, this lead support person.

In the beginning, the sufferer will need a member of the family support team in any fearful situation. When he or she gets stronger and is able to venture further without help, the support person can wait by the telephone. Later, when everything in the practice session is going well, and the sufferer has gained some self-confidence, a support person won't need to be available on a regular basis. The agoraphobic will be able to carry on alone most of the time and practice by him- or herself. If the sufferer knows one of the support team can be relied on, he or she will feel more confident in venturing forth without help. At this point, the sufferer will need much less assistance.

## What Is Good Support?

A good support person is someone who accepts the problem, has the knowledge to understand the healing process, and the patience to wait. This is an individual who is willing to help the sufferer solve his or her problems, not bury or run away from them.

Dr. Hardy liked to compare agoraphobia to a situation in which a wife has a broken leg from a skiing accident. Her husband is understanding, sympathetic, and helpful. He waits patiently for the healing process until she is well and he has his ski partner back again. That's the kind of help a support person must offer. Although the problem in this case is a mental phobia, it is just as real for the sufferer as any physical problem.

Unfortunately, relatives often have an archaic attitude because of the stigma associated with anything related to psychiatrists, psychologist, or therapy—anything related to *mental health*. "It's okay," as one support person husband said, "to tell people your wife has cancer and is taking chemotherapy, but a husband would think it bad to say his wife has agoraphobia and is therapeutically working to overcome this ailment."

What helped him deal with the disorder, not only as a spouse, but as a support person, was to approach his wife's phobic problems as a sickness, a disease that he and his wife were working on together to cure. "I took what was an unseeable problem (you can't put a cast around a phobia) and in my mind's eye visualized it as an illness. Just as most spouses wouldn't be angry with their wives if they had cancer or diabetes, why would you do so with something like phobia problems? If your wife had cancer you'd have initial pain, anger, and frustration that it happened to her and that the disease affected your lives. All the 'why me's' would hit you. But after some time you'd resolve to do something about the disease, and your feelings would lessen. You'd probably want to find out all you could about the disease and how it could be cured. You'd want to be supportive. You'd want to find out any limitations she would have and adjust your life to live as comfortably as you could with these limitations."

Aside from this, a support person must balance his or her help. In his practice, Dr. Hardy found that too much help breeds dependency and too little inhibits progress. This creates a paradox: If a support person helps too much, the sufferer becomes spoiled and wants more. It's nice to have that much attention, but it's not good for the sufferer. It is possible to become addicted to this attention. Often sufferers have so little confidence in themselves that they attach themselves to those closest to them. On the other hand, if the support person doesn't help enough, the individual suffering from agoraphobia feels abandoned. Then, thinking that no one cares, the sufferer stops trying to get better. It's important to create balance.

Let me give you an example. Dr. Hardy was treating a mother and her agoraphobic adult daughter. During a counseling session the daughter began to cry. The mother immediately reached into her purse for a Kleenex. He said to her, "No Kleenex. Let her cry. She needs to let her emotions out." He explained to the mother that her daughter wasn't in pain, she was simply emotional. Pretty soon the daughter stopped crying, her eyes cleared up, and she began to laugh. "That's funny," she told him, "I haven't really cried for five years."

This mother had always been too quick to run to her daughter's aid. The daughter's reaction to her mother's behavior became like an addiction. It's nice to have that much attention, but it can stop any possible recovery.

One family support member compared his role to helping someone change a burned out light bulb in a ceiling fixture. The burned out bulb is the problem that needs to be solved. The recovery steps are the ladder, the tool used to resolve the problem. The sufferer is the one who has to resolve the problem of changing the light bulb, climbing the ladder. The family support team is there to hold the ladder steady while she does. They are not there to push her aside and do the job themselves, or tell her how to do it. Yet they will also not walk away and leave the suffering person to struggle in the dark. They simply hold the ladder, offer encouragement, and remind the sufferer that the light is out.

Realize that you are there as a support person, but you are not there to sacrifice your life to the other person. Don't take over and do everything for the phobic. Instead, try to help this person stand on his or her own feet. To recover, it is essential for the sufferer to begin to feel a sense of his or her own identity and autonomy.

Usually the people I see have so little confidence in themselves that they want to attach themselves to those closest to them. Remember, it's important not to reinforce your afflicted loved one's dependency.

.   .   .

## Can You Be a Good Support Person?

You can be a good support person—even if you don't understand the disorder, even if the suffer's affliction sometimes makes you angry and frustrated, even if you can't believe anyone could really be afraid of things which don't look scary, and even when the disorder has made your life miserable.

You are only human and need not be perfect. However, you must give the sufferer your unconditional support. For example, in another one of Dr. Hardy's sessions with a patient and her husband, the topic of discussion was the dissension and arguments going on within the family because of the wife's disorder. When the couple first sat down, they sat apart, the wife sitting on one side of Dr. Hardy and the husband on the other. While sitting there, the husband looked at the ceiling and walls and seemed to be biding his time. Finally, he began to listen to what Dr. Hardy had to say. Suddenly he started to cry. Dr. Hardy handed him a tissue, and as the man took it he said, "I realize I've been a bad partner. I've done everything wrong. I'm just making her worse."

The next morning the couple came in holding hands. Once the spouse or other family support person accepts and opens his or her mind about the sufferer's disorder, things began to change. At this point, attitude and the way the sufferer perceives it are everything.

When family members are angry because of the disorder, sometimes it's because they fear other people will not understand the condition. This is a normal reaction. However, it's important as a support person to keep communications open by discussing any anger and fear you might have with the sufferer. It's better, as one spouse said, "to be angry and frustrated *along with* your partner than being angry and frustrated *at* him or her."

Every member of the family support team needs to keep an open mind toward the sufferer's disorder and the recovery process. This gives all of you a chance to grow and change as the person recovers.

## Types of Support People

You might think that every support person would immediately

dedicate themselves to helping the sufferer conquer his or her disorder and give unconditional support. Unfortunately, agoraphobia is one of those disorders that often catches the family by surprise. In the beginning they react in different ways. Some refuse to accept it as a legitimate disorder and deny there's anything wrong; others try to will the problem away. Still others simply become furious with the sufferer.

But remember, your overall attitude is probably the most important tool the sufferer has in his or her fight to recover. No matter where you start, you must either support the sufferer with your attitude or not be part of the family support team.

Unfortunately, throughout his years of practice Dr. Hardy saw many attitudes and actions on the part of the support team that were extremely destructive to the sufferer's effort to recover.

Here are the characteristics of some of the lead support people that he found. Each support person has a characteristic trait that is most predominant, but there are support people who do, in many ways, fit several categories.

The lead support person that is talked about can be a husband, mother, father, aunt, uncle, son or daughter—any person closely associated. But since the majority are the spouse of the sufferer, they are referred to as the "very capable spouse" and so forth. When reading about them, try to be as honest and objective about yourself as you can. The idea is to identify the unacceptable traits you see here in your own reaction so that you understand what kind of an attitude and actions you must present to help the sufferer recover.

### The Very Capable Spouse

This lead support member's capabilities appear to overshadow the sufferer. As the union develops, it tends to polarize itself, so that the more capable person (usually a spouse) becomes increasingly capable by doing more and more for the agoraphobic, while the one who has the disorder begins to feel more and more incapable.

The sufferer begins to give in to the more capable spouse, looking to him or her for guidance and direction. Gradually the sufferer gives up his or her personality, independence, self-sufficiency, self-worth, self-esteem, and self-confidence until this person is unable to know what he or she wants in the world or how to find it. Always looking for someone else to take charge, the sufferer becomes overly dependent and a burden in the relationship.

An example: When Beth, a South Carolina woman, first became ill, her husband Alan took over all her responsibilities rather than trying to help her through them. As time went on, he ended up doing more and more. And the more he did for her, the less she did for herself. She didn't get better until he stopped trying to over-help and began to let her take on more responsibilities.

Sometimes the "capable spouse" doesn't even realize what he or she is doing until it's pointed out. However, this person can learn to have a better grasp over the effect of being too capable, making efforts during recovery to consciously restrict the effort to do too much. This allows the sufferer to grow, developing his or her own capacities to their highest potential.

*The Quiet, Inhibited Spouse*

This lead team member doesn't exhibit any emotion or opinion whatsoever. This is such a contrast to the sufferer's outgoing, excitable personality that he or she begins to make an effort to curtail the outpouring of emotions. This often causes the spouse to become increasingly inhibited. The sufferer finds him- or herself holding in a great many feelings. After holding in feelings for a certain length of time, this person begins to develop physiological reactions. Very frequently phobic reactions occur at the time when some feeling that has been repressed suddenly threatens to become overt.

Sometimes this particular lead person tries to communicate more. But if he or she is shy, or having anxieties, too, it may be difficult.

A good example of this is Robert, the husband of Melissa, a sufferer in Connecticut. "My husband can't deal with my problem," Melissa told me. "It's too emotional for him. He can't handle the stress. His way of coping with it is to block everything out or totally immerse himself in a hobby so he won't have to think about problems."

How did this affect her? Because she was unable to talk with him about her affliction, it only widened the rift. "In all honesty," she told me, "I feel great resentment toward him."

Sometimes, when a quiet inhibited family member learns about a relative's fears, it brings his or her own hidden fears and anxieties to light. This was the case with Jonathan, a Dayton, Ohio, man: "I discovered, while going through the Terrap program as my wife's support person, that I had phobias and anxieties, too. They might not have been as big as my wife's, but I did become more aware of having them." As often happens, in helping his wife with recovery, Jonathan also learned to help himself.

### The Overprotective Spouse

This family member tends to infantilize the sufferer by being super-careful and excessively solicitous of the problem. As Alicia, one sufferer, told me, "My husband treats me like a child. He even withholds information that he thinks would upset me. This irritates me to no end."

The difficulty is there are secondary gains from this overly protective relationship that reinforce the sufferer's need for attention, comfort, and security. This helps to perpetuate and even exaggerate the problem. The agoraphobic loses self-confidence and self-esteem by making him- or herself submissive to the spouse. The sufferer reasons that the overprotective spouse would be disappointed if the sufferer did not need that person to watch over him or her. This complicates the recovery.

Friends can also be guilty of over-protection, as Sherie, a Royal Oaks, Michigan, sufferer, pointed out. "Although supportive," she said, "two of my women friends also tended to protect me rather than help me get over my problem." Treating the sufferer this way often prevents self-development. Support people need to realize that all adult agoraphobics must be treated as equals.

The overly protective spouse generally has greater difficulty in making changes. This person has formed a strong habit that is difficult to alter—that of wanting to care for someone to the extent of preventing his or her self-development.

## Chapter 6

### The Dictatorial Spouse

This relative tries to dominate the sufferer, which is intimidating to the agoraphobic's fragile personality. Often, the sufferer then becomes convinced that he or she can't take care of him- or herself and needs to be dominated and disciplined to continue to function on a proper level.

"To be the way my husband wants me to be, it seems like I have to do everything to please him," Jean, a sufferer in New Haven, Connecticut, said in an interview. "He seems to like me better when I behave as he wants me to. When I practice driving he wants to be in control. This makes me feel as if I'm not capable of handling it myself and increases my anxiety." In keeping with his needs, her needs were not being satisfied, slowing her progress.

Dictatorial behavior from the spouse destroys the sufferer's ability to be spontaneous and inhibits him or her drastically. When the sufferer has a spontaneous idea or desire, he or she often hesitates to act, and frequently a severe anxiety reaction occurs. There is a conflict between coming out with impulsive feelings and holding them in. The dictatorial spouse seems to have great difficulty in relinquishing the dictatorial position. He likes the power and tends to hold onto it.

### The "Put-Down Artist" or Critical Spouse

The "put-down artist" believes that the troubles of the world can be corrected by punishment. Punishment generally comes in the form of criticism and put-downs intended to correct a situation. In reality they hurt the sufferer's feelings. For example, Deidre, a woman in Santa Ana, California, said, "When my husband becomes angry because of my disorder he cuts me with words. 'It's all your fault that the family doesn't do anything together'; 'You're such a wimp'; 'I wish I had a companion to do something with.'" Even threats were not beyond him. "You're going to lose me one of these days." Nor were unsympathetic remarks, such as "Not this again. Let's just go home." All of this created even greater anxiety.

In talking to fellow sufferers I was surprised to hear many complain that their spouses put them down because of their disorder.

Larry, a Michigan man, said his wife would become angry when they were out together and his anxiety got the best of him. His affliction interfered with what she wanted to do. Larry also complained that his wife used the disorder as a weapon during arguments.

Instead of correcting the situation, criticisms and put-downs give the sufferer a sense of weakness and imperfection that the sufferer must cover up. Vivian, a Michigan woman, added that her husband's remarks had the same detrimental effect. "When my husband gets angry about anything he gives me snippy remarks. Then I have trouble going out with him because he is upset. If we are out and he gets angry, I start thinking negative things like 'What if he leaves me here'—even though, inside, I know he wouldn't." As she explained, "When agoraphobics like me have spouses who anger easily, it makes life harder, and it can take longer to recover."

The critical spouse is a put-down expert. He may do this in the guise of trying to be helpful, hoping that pointing out faults and weaknesses will correct the situation. Able to see the deleterious effects of this on the sufferer, this person may try to stop the put-downs, but they stem from a long history of hostility and dissatisfaction within. Thus, when hostility creeps into the relationship, the spouse reverts to the put-downs and criticism as a way of hurting the sufferer.

The critical person is not always the lead support person. As Jennifer, a woman from Long Beach, California, reports, "Friends and other family members can also be mean. There have been times when I would rather take a beating than hear their cruel words."

Sufferers are very sensitive. Negative remarks can have a devastating effect on their sense of well-being. "When people criticize me," Lori, another sufferer, said, "it just reinforces my own doubts about myself and lowers my confidence."

In some cases, after a sufferer begins to get help for the disorder, a relative who has not been supportive will change and begin to offer him or her some assistance. For instance, Tyler the husband of Robin, a Marysville, California, sufferer, was not supportive of his wife's efforts to recover. He was also against her seeking help for her problem. Despite his opposition, Robin entered a phobia program. Once she took the responsibility, she began to notice some positive changes in her spouse. "In the beginning, Tyler laughed and criticized me," she said. "He still does sometimes. However, he is now trying his best to overcome this attitude and be more supportive. The only problem is that, although he is trying, he really doesn't know how yet. *But at least he is trying!*"

Usually these behaviors do not change unless spouses and other relatives participate in recovery and become part of the support team. Otherwise these people may exhibit high resistance, overtly or covertly, to changing their behaviors, and they may also exhibit resistance to any changes in their suffering relative. This often leads to sabotage of the sufferer's treatment program. In situations like this, it is very helpful for these people to get outside help to treat the disorder.

Unfortunately, agoraphobia and panic disorder often create unbalanced relationships among spouses, parents, and other close companions. If conflict and tension already exist in the relationship before the disorder, then it may be advisable to avoid acting as a support person. In addition, in cases like this, to preserve the marriage and family during and after recovery, you should seek professional guidance and instruction from a clinician with expertise in both family therapy and the treatment of agoraphobia and panic disorder. If, however, the family relationship has a good foundation and the conflict and tension is because of the disorder (not other problems), you can improve the relationship by systematically working together to overcome it.

Now let's get down to the fundamentals of support and the family therapy attitude basics.

### Building a "Phobic Nest"

The instinct for survival in life requires the establishment of a nest where one is safe, secure, and sheltered from the outside elements. For instance, a while back one of Dr. Hardy's office staff acquired a new kitten. When she first brought it home it ran under the bed, but slowly it ventured out from its safe place and learned how to get to the kitchen to eat. Then the kitten began tolerating people, and it soon had the run of the house.

Much the same, before a sufferer can begin to face fears, this person must first have a safe place to which to retreat. It is a necessary part of the sufferer's recovery process.

Dr. Hardy called this safe place the "phobic nest." In this phobic nest the sufferer can get away from the harshness of the world, the crowds, the stress, the disappointments, the demands, and the pressures. This person can retreat to this place to recover from hurts, anxieties, and nervousness and know what it's like to be calm. The sufferer can also be happy here, because he or she feels loved and accepted in spite of the disorder.

The likelihood of a sufferer developing an anxiety attack while in the phobic nest is minimal, because this person learns from experience that going to and staying in this nest alleviates the symptoms of anxiety. Thus, he or she feels relatively calm and most of all secure here.

The family support team's first job is to help establish this phobic nest. However, it's important to note that the sufferer does not get well *inside* this phobic nest, only *outside* of it. But once the nest is developed, the family support team can begin to help the sufferer move away from this area of security and into the outside world—the more the sufferer recovers, the further away from the nest he or she will move, and so on.

The phobic nest consists of three main components: (1) a safe person or persons, (2) a safe place, and (3) a therapeutic climate.

*A Safe Person*

The "safe person" is an individual who is non-critical and non-judgmental of the sufferer. This person loves and accepts the sufferer just as he or she is and offers companionship and a congenial and relaxed relationship where the sufferer can feel free to express feelings. The safe person establishes and attitude of collaboration and negotiation with the sufferer. This person forms a therapeutic alliance with the sufferer, making the problem "our problem," not the sufferer's problem alone. Generally safe people are the spouse and family, and maybe one or two best friends. They are the sufferer's support people and members of the support team.

*A Safe Place*

The sufferer must have a place where he or she can get away from stress and emotional tension and feel free of his or her anxiety. This is a safe spot where the sufferer feels secure and happy, protected from any noxious outside stimuli. Here, this person can retreat from anxiety, rest, recharge his or her energy, and then go back out into the world to face his or her fears. Because the environment needs to be one the sufferer is familiar with and there needs to be an association with those people who love and accept the sufferer, this safe place is most often the sufferer's home. Sometimes it can even be a specific room in the home, such as the sufferer's bedroom.

*A Therapeutic Climate*

The sufferer's recovery can only take place in the right environment. Together the safe person(s) and the safe place create the right environment, a loving and caring atmosphere for the sufferer to get well in. This atmosphere is called the "therapeutic climate," and its overall foundation is built from proper support and the right recovery attitude on the part of the family support team.

How do support people create a therapeutic climate? Understanding, patience, and acceptance are the best approaches to healing. Dr. Hardy taught support people that acceptance means love, patience means you care, and understanding means you are willing to get to know your partner better.

Along with acceptance, patience, and understanding, there are a number of other effective components necessary to create a therapeutic climate. They include the fourteen elements necessary to be an effective support person and twenty-eight do's and don'ts that lead to recovery.

## The Fourteen Elements Necessary to Be an Effective Support Person

1. *Acceptance.* An effective support person must accept the problem from the outset. This means you accept the agoraphobic condition for what it is at this moment. Dr. Hardy found in his

practice that acceptance is an active, positive, and caring action, in contrast to nonacceptance, which is passive, negative, and often hostile. Acceptance, he said, does not mean that a person has to like what he or she accepts.

For example, you may not like the weather. If you're nonaccepting, you will become passive and complain, or you may become angry, withdrawn, and depressed. On the other hand, if you accept the weather, you can cope with it by dressing appropriately and taking a chance on being uncomfortable. You will make the best of a bad situation. Much the same, you may not like the fact that a family member suffers from agoraphobia. That's understandable. But you can learn to cope with the disorder. This is a much better approach to the problem than complaining or becoming angry.

It is not uncommon, however, for sufferers to try to hide their affliction. They often maintain a façade of being perfect by acting as if it doesn't exist. This causes them to become self-hating, complaining, depressed, and non-accepting. If they can learn to accept their disorder, they will do away with this self-hatred and become more compassionate with themselves.

The sufferer's first step is to accept him- or herself. Your most important step is to accept his or her problem.

2. *Understanding.* You must be willing to learn about the condition and help your afflicted partner understand the problem. Dr. Hardy always stressed to support people, "You must realize that you are dealing with an intense fear that makes people want to run away and hide and to resist doing things that entail risk and change."

As a support person, you need to educate yourself about the problem. This can come from a book, such as this one, a phobia treatment program, a self-help support group, or whatever. Acquire all the information you can about agoraphobia and panic disorder, then read (and re-read) the material. Bone up on the facts. This is an essential step. Before family (or even friends) can help, they need to have a clear understanding of what the disorder really means. Without this knowledge, they'll feel as if an unknown horror is waiting, ready to strike when they least expect it.

3. *Sincerity.* You must truly want to see the sufferer recover. Be sincere when you offer to help. Be sincere when you show him

or her how pleased you are that the agoraphobic is making some gains toward recovery. Care about the sufferer's welfare and how the disorder has affected his or her life.

4. *Compassion (Kindness).* Try to have a sense of the suffering the phobic has been going through. Be sympathetic of the difficulties. A kind word, a gentle touch, a smile, or an understanding look can do a great deal to lessen the sufferer's anxiety.

5. *Enouragement.* Recovery is a one-step-at-a-time process. You need to encourage the sufferer to continue forward on a regular basis and to adopt a "don't give up" attitude. Point out the progress that the sufferer has made. Give encouragement in small, frequent doses and, above all, make it sincere.

6. *Readiness.* A support person needs to show a readiness to do what is helpful—the fact that you are reading this book means you have taken a very important step. If the sufferer is enrolled in a recovery program or self-help group and you are attending the meetings as a support person, all the better.

7. *Patience.* Improvement is not steady; it comes in waves. Sometimes progress will be slow. The sufferer can recover, but it will take time for the mind and body to learn new reactions and thought patterns. This process cannot be rushed.

Everyone learns at their own pace. Whether it be a new skill like riding a bike, an activity like bowling or tennis, or the three Rs—reading, writing, and arithmetic—it is human nature that different people learn at different speeds. Since the recovery steps are also a learning process, one cannot expect all sufferers to progress at the same level. Therefore, patience from you is vital. Make allowances for whatever pace the sufferer finds most comfortable. Permit the agoraphobic to make mistakes, then help the sufferer to learn from them. Encourage him or her to try again.

8. *Tolerance.* Tolerance is a close cousin of acceptance. People who are tolerant accept others just as they are, in spite of their faults and weaknesses. Be tolerant of your afflicted loved one's behavior. Try not to think of the phobic fears and avoidance as weird. Above all, do not turn away. Remember, this behavior is caused by a temporary anxiety disorder. As the sufferer improves, so will the behavior.

9. *Recognition.* It is important for you to reward any accomplishments made during recovery. Remember that no one who has agoraphobia and panic disorder wants to have it. The sufferer wants to recover, but recovery requires effort. Sufferers need a direction. They will put out the effort, providing there is some payoff. A short-term payoff such as praise, a reward, recognition, or affection from support people can be most helpful and motivating.

The ideal reward is one that comes from within the sufferer when he or she feels good about the accomplishments. However, verbal strokes from the support person, especially in the beginning, can make a great deal of difference.

In clinical observation, Dr. Hardy discovered that small rewards are much more motivating than threats, punishment, or criticism. Avoid criticism, put-downs, threats, demands, and yelling. These methods only aggravate the problem and cause the phobic person to close up. Instead, encourage the sufferer's practice with rewards. For example, you might tell him or her: "When you are able to go out to a restaurant, let's celebrate by eating somewhere very special."

Since regular practice is so important, compliment the sufferer on his or her consistent practice and on *any* progress made—sufferers need praise for even the smallest steps.

10. *Trustworthiness.* The sufferer must trust you and feel secure in your presence. Remember, you are dealing with fear. People with agoraphobia and panic disorder are extremely insecure, very sensitive, easily frightened, and lacking in self-confidence. They have little assurance in their own capabilities.

How do you gain trust? Sit down as a support team and discuss the individual role each of you will have in the recovery process. Ask the sufferer what he or she expects from each of you and in what way you can best help. Also ask how he or she feels about the disorder and the recovery process. In Chapter 11, I discuss this initial meeting and subsequent practice session meetings and detail what should be discussed at each. I will also give you some guidelines to follow.

The sufferer must build trust in you before building confidence in his or her own ability to manage. Do not make promises you can't keep. This is imperative. If you say, "I will meet you in ten minutes," *be there,* or don't promise at all.

11. *Responsibility.* Recognize the sufferer is responsible for his or her own recovery. Even though you are giving your support, the problem itself lies with the phobic person. Only he or she can decide when to get better. Just as there is no magic pill that will make the problem disappear, no outside person can cure the one who suffers. You must let the sufferer take the lead.

It is the sufferer's responsibility to tell you when the anxiety has subsided, when the practice session is over, or when you are no longer needed for support. This allows him or her to feel more independence. It also allows you to have more freedom and choice over your support role and still retain a close relationship with the sufferer.

It is the sufferer's responsibility for the way in which he or she handles phobic situations. He or she is also responsible for the pace. As a support person, you are there only to guide and assist, to give encouragement and protection when needed, to oversee recovery, to offer suggestions, and to remind the sufferer of the behavioral skills he or she has learned.

12. *Speak the language.* Learn to speak the phobic's language. The recovery process has a language all its own. This language is universal, as most treatment programs and phobia books use the same or similar words. This way, when your partner begins to talk about practicing, about number 3s and number 10s, about desensitization and fallacious beliefs, self-talk and feelings, you will understand and be able to discuss these things.

13. *Modeling.* Be a model for your partner. Show your partner how to act. For example, the sufferer is always controlled by his or her negative anticipation. The most effective way for the sufferer to change a thinking pattern is to associate with people who have a more positive pattern of thinking. Since you are probably closest to the sufferer, maintain a positive attitude about the disorder and life in general; he or she will pick up on this and learn new ways of coping with the world. (Some tips on how to maintain a positive attitude appear later in this book.)

Psychologist Albert Bandura at Stanford University treated

snake phobias by using the modeling technique. He would first let the phobic person watch the instructor handle the snake, then ask the fearful person to touch it.

14. *Participation.* Actively participate in the agoraphobic's recovery. Jerilyn Ross recommends that spouses or other support people attend phobia treatment programs along with their phobic partners. She says, "Most studies show, when a family team works together to overcome agoraphobia and panic disorder, it strengthens the sufferer's marriage and the extended family and makes the therapeutic recovery process better."

Sufferers require a great deal of backing and reinforcement, especially in the beginning. When your suffering partner embarks upon a self-improvement project, you can help or you can sabotage. Dr. Hardy said, "Indifference is sabotage. Making partners do it alone is inconsiderate. Hindering partners' progress is cruelty. Putting the sufferer down is sadism. Understanding is loving. Doing it for the phobic is impossible. And *support* is caring."

## Twenty-Eight Do's and Don'ts That Lead to Recovery

To help you achieve positive attitude growth here is a list of universal factors that lead to recovery. Because of the nature of their importance, you will see many of these items repeated in one form or another throughout the book.

### *Do's*

1. *Praise always.* Normal activities that might seem insignificant to others, such as eating in a restaurant, driving a car, attending a party, or even walking down the street, take a great deal of work and much courage for the sufferer to perform.

Compliment any and all of the sufferer's positive steps toward improvement. Always make mountains out of molehills. This will help him or her venture into more challenging situations in the future. However, only acknowledge true progress.

2. *Make plans for your recovery activities.* Plan the activities you will be doing together and the activities each will be expected to do separately.

Help the sufferer set short-range goals and work with him or her on these goals. For example, before the practice session in which the sufferer is going to be confronting a situation that he or she has been avoiding, plan ahead of time what it you are going to face, how you are going to approach the situation, and what recovery tools you will both be using. The final decision about what he or she will face and the specific recovery steps will always be the sufferer's decision. However, it is helpful to have someone to talk with about any feelings and concerns.

3. *Share feelings.* The sharing of feelings brings team members closer. Don't keep your feelings bottled up; be open. Encourage the sufferer to do the same. Share any concerns you have about the disorder and the recovery process. Sharing is an avenue by which togetherness is reached. When you share feelings, intimate thoughts, fantasies, and secrets, you become closer.

If you really want to get to know the sufferer, you must risk letting him or her get to know you. Talk as you would to a friend, with humor, understanding, tolerance, and interest. Talking and sharing experiences and feelings is the best way to truly know one another. This takes time, so allow each other this gift.

4. *Respect feelings.* Respect is always of high importance. Respect the sufferer's feelings, even if you don't agree with or understand them. Let the sufferer know it's okay to express feelings, for the expression of feelings is a sign of improvement.

Also let the sufferer know it's okay to cry. (Since this is a form of expression many men don't use, this is especially important if the sufferer is a man.) Crying offers a release of tension.

5. *Give choices.* Encourage the sufferer's freedom of choice. Let him or her decide what to practice and when he or she needs to practice with you. Let the sufferer tell you when the practice session is over.

Never ask the sufferer to do something he or she can't do. The sufferer needs to feel in control. Freedom of choice gives control over the situation and over his or her own life. This builds the sufferer's confidence in you as a support person and in him- or herself, which in turn builds trust and independence.

Instead of suggesting changes yourself, ask the sufferer to

access what changes he or she wants. Keep these small to begin with. For example, if the sufferer is a woman and you always shop with her, ask her how she thinks she could alter the procedure for her own benefit. Perhaps she will tell you to wait for her at the cash register, at the door, or in the car. Or perhaps, for variety, she would rather try this activity with another person. It doesn't matter how she changes the activity; the important part is that she changes to a *less secure* situation.

6. *Give attention.* The disorder has caused the sufferer to lose self-confidence and self-esteem, so let the sufferer know he or she is important and worthwhile. Point out good qualities.

7. *Show affection.* Love brings out the best in people, physically, emotionally, and spiritually. Don't overlook the physical expression of feelings. It helps to soften the hard realities of life.

Any time you show affection it is appreciated, and sooner or later it will be returned. Remember, the agoraphobic's disorder has made him or her feel insecure and sometimes even unworthy of love and affection. A show of affection, such as a hug, goes much further than a lot of words. If you see that the agoraphobic is frightened in a situation, your hug or handhold will go much further in relieving stress than all the lectures in the world.

8. *Show the importance of problems and their resolution.* Offer your help; don't wait to be asked. Remind the sufferer how important recovery is to you and how much fuller and better both your lives can be when he or she has recovered. Remind the sufferer that with this recovery program there is a chance of overcoming the problem.

Take the time to work through any difficulties the sufferer may be having because of the disorder. Don't give up on problems; follow them through to their resolution. Persistence pays off!

9. *Show appreciation for the sufferer and the sufferer's efforts.* Appreciation goes hand in hand with encouragement and praise. This common courtesy builds good will between you and the sufferer. Any compliment you give, no matter how small, is a positive step toward the sufferer's improvement. Remember, sufferers lack self-confidence. They have little faith in themselves and their own abilities. If you show the sufferer that you appreciate his or her efforts to

recover, it rebuilds self-confidence destroyed by the disorder.

10. *Show confidence in the agoraphobic's ability to handle things.* This also builds the sufferer's self-confidence, which in turn helps the individual become more independent and self-reliant.

Sufferers often believe that they can't cope with much of anything. In spite of this, you should avoid stepping in and doing things for them. This reinforces their feelings of weakness and helplessness.

11. *Encourage spontaneity.* As the sufferer begins to improve and become more self-confident, encourage him or her to be more spontaneous. Encouraging spontaneity will help remove inhibitions.

12. *Encourage positive thinking.* This will help the sufferer deal with the down periods and get to the up periods sooner. It's also important for you as a family support member to let go of feelings of anger, disappointment, or resentment about the disorder.

*Don'ts*

1. *Don't force by any method.* Force is defeating. If you pressure the agoraphobic to do something before he or she is ready, you prevent progress.

Carla, one spouse with whom I spoke, forced her afflicted husband Tim into situations that brought on his panic attacks, then insisted he stay there until the panic went away. This only made him worse.

When Carla began to *encourage* him instead of forcing him, he started to improve. As Tim said in an interview, "I think this is the reason I finally dared venture out and do things." Carla's new approach let him remain in total control. He no longer felt forced to stay in a situation that made him uncomfortable. Consequently, he was able to risk being there.

2. *Don't compare to others.* Never compare the sufferer to other people. It is a fact of human nature that everyone is different. Comparison not only hurts because it is negative; it is also an invitation for the sufferer to dislike him- or herself.

In *Pulling Your Own Strings,* Dr. Wayne W. Dyer said, "In a world of individuals, comparison is a senseless activity."

Comparison, he believes, is just a meaningless way people have of manipulating someone to do what they think is best for that person, not what that person thinks is best for him- or herself.

3. *Don't placate or make excuses.* You should never give in to the sufferer's demands or make excuses for him or her. When a team member makes excuses for the sufferer all the time, it separates them and tends to retard progress.

4. *Don't criticize other than constructively.* Negative criticism is lethal. We all have faults. Don't bring up the sufferer's faults unless you are willing to hear your own. Daily recitation of faults doesn't make things better; it only tends to convince the sufferer that he or she is unworthy.

Because the sufferer is already lacking in self-confidence and self-esteem, the only time you should correct him or her is when you are helping the sufferer learn a new recovery skill. If you must criticize, do it constructively and keep your words kind.

5. *Don't be judgmental or labeling.* Eliminate any tendency you may have to assess and evaluate. Sufferers are their own worst critics. Sufferers don't need someone else to evaluate what they already think is their own reality.

6. *Don't sabotage the recovery program—it works.* Every sufferer is entitled to a chance at recovery. Even if you are doubtful about some of the recovery steps, give the family support system—or whatever recovery program the sufferer has chosen—a chance. You just may find that it works.

Do not attempt to change any of the recovery steps because you think something else might work better. And encourage the sufferer to adhere to them.

7. *Don't make assumptions.* Don't suddenly become innovative. If the sufferer has planned to go one block, don't assume two or three blocks would be better. No surprises. Stay with the original plan.

8. *Don't solve problems for the sufferer.* The sufferer needs to be in charge of his or her own life and recovery. To become independent and self-reliant, sufferers must learn to solve their own problems. Help only by suggesting options. Include everyone connected with the problem: children or other close relatives.

Offer the sufferer all the help you can give, but remember that only he or she can do it. If he or she avoids running an errand, don't offer to run it yourself. Instead, offer to accompany the sufferer on the errand with the understanding that if the agoraphobic becomes anxious and can't complete it, you will.

9. *Don't be overly concerned.* Don't walk on eggshells. The sufferer can handle quite a bit despite his or her complaints, anger, frustration, etc. Remember to think of yourself, too; otherwise neither of you will grow.

10. *Don't psychoanalyze.* Some of the information in this book is psychological in nature. Information like this is easy to misuse. Sufferers do not want advice; they want understanding. Be a support person, but don't try to psychoanalyze your afflicted loved one.

11. *Don't preach.* Eliminate the words *should* and *shouldn't* from your vocabulary. Let the sufferer decide what he or she should and shouldn't do. This builds self-confidence and independence.

Never lecture about the problem or the length of time the recovery is taking. This accomplishes nothing.

12. *Don't surprise with unexpected company or trips.* No surprises! The sufferer likes to be in control *at all times.* The first rule of good interpersonal relationships is not to make any plans that involve the sufferer without including him or her in the planing.

13. *Don't ridicule.* Ridicule is a terrorist tactic. It undermines recovery. Don't ridicule, demand, threaten separation, ignore, or use the silent treatment to gain power over the sufferer. This lowers self-esteem and self-confidence.

14. *Don't set time limits.* For the sufferer to overcome the disorder, he or she must be allowed to set the pace. Patience is difficult when you are tired of living with the problem, but recovery is made by three steps forward and one step back. Pushing the sufferer only prevents progress!

15. *Don't question the sufferer's progress.* This only makes the phobic worry about not progressing fast enough. Instead, let the sufferer volunteer information.

16. *Never withhold physical affection to punish.* Family support people should frequently hug and touch the sufferer. Drawing back makes the phobic unsure. In addition, the spouse should not withhold

sex as punishment. Sex is not a weapon, nor is it a way to negotiate. Sex should be given in love and enjoyed in trust.

## THE MOST IMPORTANT THING YOU CAN DO

The most important thing you can do for the sufferer is to *never give up.* I can't stress enough how important that is. Mike Ditka, the former head coach of the Chicago Bears football team, once said, "You never lose until you stop trying." The only way your loved one will lose the battle to recover is if he or she stops trying to conquer the disorder.

Don't give up on yourself as a support person. Stay with it, especially when times seem to be bleakest. Remember, you are not alone. When you know in advance what problems to expect, you have a better handle on how to deal with them if and when they arrive. Not only does this knowledge help build your confidence as a support person, but every time you tackle a problem and are victorious, the sufferer will come a step closer to conquering his or her disorder.

The more experienced you become with these problems, the better you will become at handling them. As Aristotle said, "People become house builders through building houses, harp players through playing the harp. We grow to be just by doing things that are just." In this same vein you can become a good support person by getting behind the sufferer and by helping support him or her with the proper attitude and actions every step of the way.

## CHAPTER SEVEN

# Building a Circle of Support

*"Clapping with the right hand only will not produce noise."*

*—Malay proverb*

Successful supported recovery need only involve one person. However, it's often difficult for a single person to meet all the sufferer's support needs. Many experts believe that the larger the circle of support, the better sufferers and their support people are able to cope with stress and the happier and healthier they will be. Adding a network of support to a recovery plan will have a multitude of benefits, enhancing the whole process immensely.

## ENLARGING THE CIRCLE OF SUPPORT

The overall circle of support includes a personal circle of support, self-support, side support people, alternate supporters, self-help support groups, and support by mail. Let's look at each of these individually.

### The Personal Circle of Support

As we grow up, if we are fortunate, we slowly build within our lives a support system that includes more than simply our parents and others in our immediate family. As time goes on, through building relationships with others we expand our network of support to include people such as other relatives (grandparents, aunts, uncles, and cousins), friends, neighbors, co-workers, associates, and other acquaintances—teachers, baby-sitters, and so on. Our support system allows us to have a variety of people in our lives who meet our various needs.

While going through the Terrap program I learned that everyone needs to build a support system in which they can feel emotionally secure, knowing there are people to meet their needs and to give and receive love and affection.

An overall support system should include the following.

1. A very special person to whom one can be very close. A special person with whom to share private, personal feelings and thoughts and still be accepted.

2. Several close relatives or friends that one sees frequently, people with whom to share almost all feelings and thoughts.

3. Approximately eight to ten good friends, people to talk to and share some thoughts and feelings with.

4. Other friends to do things with. These are people to socialize with, play golf or go places with, and so on. One may associate with these people but not share the same closeness as with the previous group of friends.

5. The rest of one's acquaintances, including all the others with whom one comes into contact in daily life: sales clerks, bank tellers, grocery checkers, the mailman, and so on.

Optimally every person has control over their own support system and can move people from one level to another. It is also common for most people to have some empty areas in their support system from time to time. However, for a person's support system to be complete, Dr. Hardy believed all of the areas should be filled.

Following the model above, on a blank sheet of paper, list your own current system of support from 1 to 5. This will show you the empty areas and give you suggestions.

. . .

## Self-Support

Sometimes, in the midst of the day-to-day trauma associated with being a support person to one with agoraphobia and panic disorder, it seems impossible to keep your own wishes, goals, and sense of fulfillment alive. Yet the more difficult the disorder makes things, the more important it is for you to maintain your own life. In the long run, it will make you a better support person.

When faced with a loved one's disorder you can let the situation overwhelm you, or you can find ways to cope. Coping with the problem is a way for you to put your life back into your own hands as well as help the sufferer. In addition, when you constructively cope with a situation, you resolve it sooner.

Here are fifteen suggestions for self-support, which will help you cope with your role as the main support person.

1. Have some outside interests of your own. Participate in activities you enjoy, such as playing golf, visiting with friends, or pursuing a hobby. It's important to have time for yourself so you can relax and recuperate. It helps when you temporarily withdraw, putting the situation out of your mind.

2. Maintain social contact with people you enjoy. Friends are a wonderful alliance, for it helps to talk out problems with a *trusted* person. Experts say that people who can openly discuss their deepest feelings with close friends are more resistant to stress.

3. Accept the limits of what you can do. You are not expected to be there to satisfy all your suffering loved one's needs all of the time. Remember, you are only human; sometimes you will be able to give more than at other times.

4. Realize your inner resources are greater than you think. Have faith in yourself and your abilities. Think of past troubles, crises, and disappointments you've weathered.

5. Accept the reality of your loved one's disorder and the limitations it creates without placing blame on yourself or others. Blame makes things worse.

6. Expect life will sometimes be unpredictable, and keep your expectations based in reality. Being realistic about the complexity of the disorder is half the battle.

7. Face problems head-on. The more you sweep problems under the rug, the less likely they are to get better. Work on one problem at a time. Decide which problems require priority and start there. Remain flexible; if the first solution doesn't work, try another approach.

8. Remember you are not alone; just knowing others have the same problem can make you feel better. Join a support group of others in the same situation, even if the sufferer doesn't attend one. If there's none in your area, consider starting one. Also, help others like yourself; you will gain much more than you give.

9. Don't be afraid to ask for assistance. Everyone needs help sometimes. For example, if the sufferer cannot be left alone and you need time away, have a friend or relative stay with him or her. One or two hours of free time can be a lifesaver.

10. Don't be afraid to seek out professional help from an anxiety disorder specialist. Some problems can be too big to handle alone. Are your efforts to deal with the problem failing to resolve it? Have you tried all the coping strategies only to find they aren't working? Realizing professional help is necessary does not mean you are weak; rather it can be a sign of strength. A couple of sessions can often put problems in a better perspective.

11. Maintain good physical and mental health. This will increase your tolerance of stress. Get sufficient exercise (it lets off steam) and follow a nutritional diet. Reduce your level of stress by employing some of the recovery techniques, such as relaxation and self-talk. Keep a journal; writing down your thoughts and feelings can be an emotional release.

12. Pay attention to how you react to stress. It's not the stress so much that causes problems; it's how one reacts.

13. Be objective about your situation. Look at the problem as if it were someone else's. How could this person make things better, and what things must this person accept? On one sheet of paper list the things you *can* do something about. On another sheet, list the things you *cannot* change. Then keep the first list and throw the second one away. From the remaining list, jot down the things (big and small) that need to be done to remedy the situation. Divide this list in two parts: what needs to be done now and what can wait.

Work on the small, easy items that need to be accomplished first. The more you accomplish, the less stressed you will feel.

14. Seek spiritual nourishment. When under stress, it helps to have the concept of a higher power. Even those who don't believe in God can still be helped by believing in a power greater than their own. The powerful love of a friendship, for example, can override the pain a person is feeling.

15. Work at remaining positive. Be optimistic, approaching all situations in a positive manner. This is a more effective way. Expect everything will go well, and it probably will.

### Friendly Support

Friends are an important part of any support system. This type of support helps to buffer stresses and make them more tolerable. With the right people there to let you know you're not alone, you'll find that you will be able to endure much more.

Here are some tips for developing and adding to this part of the support system:

· Take action. Go on an intentional search for friends. If you meet with rejection—which we all do at times—move onward. Eventually someone will respond to your efforts.

· Continually make new acquaintances; don't let age be a barrier. Use your own favorite interests to meet people whose company you might enjoy. For example, if you are a golfer, the driving range is a likely place to make a new friend. If you're interested in art, take an art class. Be creative in this search.

· Ask other people to join you in enjoying an established interest you usually do alone: your daily walk, going to a play, enjoying a concert, and so forth.

· Become an active member of a church or organization. Not only will you meet new people, but this will give you social activities to attend as well.

· Smile when you meet and talk to people. It's a simple but wonderful way to make a good first impression.

· Look for the good rather than the bad in people, and avoid criticizing others. When expressing yourself, be positive rather than negative, reflecting optimism instead of pessimism. Give the impression that you enjoy life and that you have a good sense of humor.

· When you meet a candidate for friendship, become genuinely interested in what that person does. Encourage people to talk about themselves.

· Let your body language say you want to be friends. Keep arms and legs uncrossed. An open body posture conveys a welcoming appearance. Maintain eye contact. This attention expresses interest and makes people feel respected.

· When people speak, lean toward them. This conveys that you are interested in them and what they have to say. People appreciate knowing you're interested. Reach out and touch someone. A heartfelt handshake, a pat on the back, or a cordial hug affirms friendship and goodwill.

· Keep relationships with the friends you have in good standing, even those you don't regularly see. When one of the areas in your own life support system becomes empty—due to lack of interest, someone moving, death, or whatever—you will have others who can fill that void.

## Side Support

Side supporters are close relatives and friends who are members of the family support team: immediate family, adult brothers and sisters, parents, children, in-laws, and even close family friends.

Side supporters help by giving emotional and physical support. Physical support means helping the sufferer do the shopping or run other errands and assisting during practice sessions, alternating with the main support person.

"Having more than one support person available to drive me," said Jill, a West Virginia woman, "is what helped me get out of the house more. It also gave me more opportunity to perform my recovery exercises."

Side supporters can also babysit children so the sufferer and the main support person can attend a recovery treatment program, therapy, or a self-help support group. They can fill in when the main support person can't attend, or they can be available to transport children or stay with a sufferer who is unable to be alone. They can make themselves available for the sufferer to reach by telephone. And, since talking about fears helps the sufferer lower his or her level of stress, somewhat easing the agoraphobia, side supporters can be available as another pair of ears ready to listen. Primarily, however, side support people help make family life as normal as possible under the circumstances.

"It helps so much when relatives and friends let us talk about feelings and fears and truly listen," John, a man from Nevada, explained. "Being able to open up to my support people when I was depressed without having them get mad and frustrated with me was a great help."

## Alternate Supporters

Besides side support people, it helps to have alternate supporters. Often these are fellow sufferers or paid para-professionals who are recovered agoraphobics. Extra support people give the sufferer added opportunities to practice recovery techniques and are available when main support people and side supporters are busy. Being kindred spirits, they sometimes work even better than relatives or friends.

As Mary Jo, a West Virginia sufferer, said, "My sister was my main support person, but she worked full-time and went to college in the evening, so her time was limited. However, I met a fellow sufferer through my recovery program, and we supported one another. I not only found an alternate support person, but was able to be one myself." In helping each other, the two of them found they were able to venture further together than if they relied on only their regular support people.

*Finding an Alternate Support Person*

There are many places to find alternate support people. Here are the best sources:

*Self-Help Support Groups.* These groups usually maintain well-publicized telephone numbers. Check the local yellow pages. Also check referral directories published by local service agencies and church bulletins and directories.

*Local Mental Health Agencies and Mental Health Associations.* They often publish a list of self-help groups, or their public information department can refer you elsewhere. Check also with the director of the local hospital's community outreach program. All can be reached through the yellow pages.

*The Psychology, Sociology, or Nursing Departments of Nearby Colleges.* They may be able to help find student support people available for schooling purposes or for a small fee. Contact the individual departments; if they can't help they may refer you to someone who can. Beth, one woman who used a recruited student for her support person, said, "We were both great help to one another. The student was supportive as I worked on different goals, and I became a teacher, explaining about agoraphobia and the recovery techniques." In the process they became close friends.

*Local Therapists.* Those who specialize in treating agoraphobia and panic disorder can often recommend a support person available either voluntarily or for pay. Again, check the yellow pages.

*Local Volunteer Bureaus.* They also maintain a list of people willing to provide a variety of services, either voluntarily or for a small fee.

*Local and Specialty (Health-Related) Newspapers.* Place an add in the classified or personals section. The advertisement could read:

NEED VOLUNTEER TO ACT AS ALTERNATE SUPPORT PERSON FOR SPOUSE WHILE (HE/SHE) PERFORMS IN-VIVO DESENSITIZATION FIELDWORK. PREFER RECOVERED AGORAPHOBIC. REFERENCES REQUIRED. PLEASE CALL ——— OR WRITE ——— FOR MORE INFO.

When using this method be sure to check all references.

*The National Self-help Group Network.* This group is sponsored by the Anxiety Disorder Association of America, 6000 Executive Blvd., Suite 513, Rockville, MD 20852-3801, (301) 231-9350. It is limited to self-help groups that specifically deal with anxiety, phobias, and related disorders. Their network directory lists over two hundred phobia self-help groups nationwide. They publish a self-help group newsletter and a guide to help you organize a phobia self-help group. In addition, they act as a key link between people and groups interested in the self-help movement.

*Other Self-Help Clearinghouses.* Sometimes other self-help clearinghouses can help. Two of them are The American Self-Help Clearinghouse, 25 Pocono Road, St. Clare's–Riverside Medical Center, Denville, NJ 07834, (201) 625-7101; and The National Self-Help Clearinghouse, City University of New York, 33 West 42nd Street, New York, NY 10036, (212) 840-1259.

## *Preparing for the Use of Alternate and Side Support People*

If you wish to add side or alternate support people to the recovery process, you must first explain to the sufferer their benefits. You might start by saying that with extra support he or she will have more opportunity to practice the recovery techniques and recover faster. You could also explain that with added support there will be someone available for him or her to call on when you are not around. Explain, too, that the more support people, the easier recovery will be on both of you. In addition, if you recruit a recovered agoraphobic to help, this person will know what the sufferer is going through and may be able to help in ways you are unable to.

Also, discuss how the sufferer prefers to approach potential support people—through you or on his or her own. Offer suggestions, but again, remember the decision rests with this person. If the sufferer is against involving anyone else, don't despair. This could change as he or she begins to recover and starts building some self-confidence.

## *Define Your Level of Involvement*

Not everyone has the disposition to be a support person. For example, Dale has a take-charge personality. This made it difficult for him to go slow enough to support his wife Audry, who was taking small but significant recovery steps. During practice sessions he became irritated and frustrated, showing little patience for Audry's needs. As a result, she began to feel like a failure and, in turn, became more withdrawn. They soon realized that practice sessions put too much strain on both of them and that Audry would be better off obtaining support elsewhere.

Others may want to offer support but can't take the time due to work or other obligations. Some people may not want to be involved at all. In such cases it's best for the sufferer that they not be, for support can't be forced.

Even those who do want to help don't always want to be fully committed to practice sessions. Many, however, are willing to offer emotional support. Even this level of support can be useful for the sufferer.

As a potential support person, you must recognize your own limitations, knowing what you are capable of tolerating in relation to the support process. Try to identify the things you feel you *can* and *cannot* do. Discuss them openly and honestly with the sufferer, so alternative solutions can be found where needed.

If you're not sure you can give the type of support necessary but are willing to try, say so. If you feel it is too much of a task to tackle alone and you want help, let the sufferer know. And if you find you either cannot or do not want to be a support person, realize this should not mean leaving the sufferer high and dry with no support. It *should* mean giving the sufferer as much emotional support as possible, while helping this person to find the needed support elsewhere.

### Self-Help Support Groups

Fortunately, support is available in many areas of the country for both the sufferer and the support person through phobia self-help support groups. In the last few years these groups have taken an active leadership role in the treatment of agoraphobia and panic disorder. Sufferers have gone from being victims who submissively receive treatment to knowledgeable consumers who actively take the lead in their own recovery. Group support gives these people the inner strength to face their fears and eventually overcome them. Strength comes in numbers.

While the main focus of phobia self-help support groups is on the sufferer, many now have separate support groups for spouses or other close relatives or allow these people to attend with the sufferer.

Self-help groups can be helpful to support people by educating them and by planting a seed of hope. For support people whose loved one is not ready to recover, a group helps maintain sanity.

Self-help support groups are also an excellent way to complement therapy and counseling. Since they are a good place to get referrals, they can even pave the way for this help.

## *Choosing a Good Support Group*

There are peer-led self-help groups and professionally run self-help groups. Both focus on group support to deal with and overcome the disorder. Both share information about the condition, emphasizing the necessity of sufferers to confront their fears, along with the importance of using coping strategies to lower anxiety levels. In both, group members find encouragement.

Professionally guided groups offer the following:

· counseling for sufferers as well as for family members who have been affected by the condition (for a fee)
· professional training in behavioral and cognitive techniques
· regularly updated information about the disorder and how to recover
· help in obtaining medication when needed
· reasonable assurance that the sufferer is getting competent treatment.

Phobia self-help support groups should offer:

· continually updated information about the disorder and the problems associated with it
· an explanation of the how-to recovery steps
· the wisdom gained from overcoming personal struggles with the disorder
· a list of the most commonly used medications and a recommendation that new members check with their doctors regarding their use
· an atmosphere of empathy, understanding, and confidentiality
· a positive approach to recovery.

·   ·   ·

They should also:

- promote the use of cognitive/behavioral procedures and relaxation techniques to confront fears; encourage sufferers to practice facing their fears outside the group and provide group practice sessions; teach sufferers to set and keep recovery goals; stay peer-led, with members sharing some responsibility for maintaining the group; include spouses or other support people directly or by providing them a separate place to meet simultaneously; and remain focused on the behavioral problems of the disorder, not personal problems.
- be free or charge a small participation fee on an ability to pay basis; have an informal "open door" policy whereby members can join and leave in accordance with their needs; and promote camaraderie and group help.
- be an adjunct to professional treatment with no one person playing the role of therapist; *not* be run as "encounter" or "therapy" group.

Membership in a self-help support group rises and falls, and the leadership changes from time to time. Always attend several meetings before making a decision as to its quality and stability.

Sufferers have recovered using the phobia self-help support group method. However, these members must have strong self-determination, along with patience and the ability to work very hard. Since it is difficult for many sufferers to take part in a support group unless they have had prior professional treatment, many experts believe self-help groups work best when used as an accompaniment or as a follow up to treatment.

Self-help support groups can be a tremendous help for many sufferers and their support people. They are also an excellent avenue for telephone support. Some provide daytime or twenty-four-hour hotline service. Some also provide transportation to and from meetings. And some visit the housebound, informing them on what it takes to recover.

However, self-help support groups can only do so much. As Meg McGarrah, Director of the Anxiety Disorder Association's Self-Help Group Network Project, said, "They can point you in the right direction and provide supportive therapy, medications can sometimes control symptoms, and a group can lend support, but you [the sufferer] alone are responsible for your recovery."

## Support by Mail

Newsletters provide up-to-date medical news and articles on agoraphobia, panic disorder, and the recovery process, including current research and the latest advances in treatment. Some offer a "pen pal" section and a special section for support people. Others offer booklets and brochures, audio and video tapes, and other informational sources about agoraphobia and panic disorder.

You will find a list of available newsletters in the Appendix.

Always use as many avenues of support as possible. That way both you and your loved one, along with members of the immediate family, can surround yourselves with a protective wall that will help to buffer the negative aspects of agoraphobia and panic disorder.

# Understanding Emotional Needs

> *"Every person's feelings have a front door and*
> *a side door by which they may be entered."*
>
> —*Oliver Wendell Holmes, Sr.*

When sufferers start to work on their disorder and have success facing their fears, they gradually let go of inhibitions. This slowly releases unfamiliar emotions and feelings, causing sufferers to become confused or frightened. When this happens, sufferers frequently believe they are getting worse when actually these feelings are often a sign of improvement.

Support people should understand this and also be aware that during recovery they will be dealing with many feelings—those of the sufferer as well as their own. Let's take a closer look at these feelings.

## BASIC HUMAN FEELINGS

The only difference between the feelings of one individual and those of another is the intensity. Feelings and emotions often translate into energy, which can be used constructively to plan a trip, dig in the garden, clean the garage, and so on. On the other hand, people who hold feelings in are often depressed, tired, or sluggish and have little energy.

## Chapter 8

While we can suppress and deny feelings, we cannot turn them off and on at will. Feelings run on automatic pilot and can be aroused by thoughts, memories, and imagination, as well as the five senses. They can also be aroused by body symptoms.

Feelings influence what we think, say, and do and can interfere with logic and reasoning. Feelings can also be transferred from one individual to another. For example, if a husband comes home feeling depressed or angry, a sensitive wife can pick up on this and feel the same way. Or if he is enthusiastic, she can "catch" his exuberant spirit. Sufferers are especially likely to absorb the feelings of others.

Feelings affect body and mind, causing a total body reaction. When we feel excited, our heart and respiration rates increase. When we feel stressed, our muscles tighten. And when we feel frightened or anxious, as in the emotional state of a panic attack, we can have all of these symptoms and more.

When sufferers hold in their feelings, they create psychological and physiological symptoms. For example, those who chronically inhibit their feelings have muscle tension. Some experts believe the location of muscle tension can be identified with different feelings—anger with the neck and shoulder muscles, sadness and grief with the muscles around the eyes and chest, fear in the stomach and intestine, and so on. Psychosomatic symptoms such as ulcers, colitis, headaches, and high blood pressure can also be caused by repressed feelings, as can free-floating anxiety unrelated to any specific circumstance. In addition, depression is often caused by repressed anger against others or oneself, or by grief or sadness.

Feelings, however, are neither good nor bad, right or wrong; they just exist. Feelings can almost always coexist and combine with other feelings such as love and anger, which in turn can create guilt.

Agoraphobics have the same feelings as any other human being, except theirs are stronger and tend to trigger more easily. To protect themselves from their intense feelings, agoraphobics often hide from them, deny them, or hold them in. To do so they usually avoid issues that bring out bad feelings.

A person's mind and body cannot distinguish one feeling from another; both encounter feelings and react to them. Thus, in holding back unpleasant feelings, sufferers often hold back pleasant feelings as well. This sometimes makes it impossible for sufferers to identify their true feelings and/or to express them. In preventing the automatic expression of natural feelings, the sufferer's tension builds until the person's body and mind can no longer take the pressure. When he or she reaches an explosion point, the body strongly overreacts, producing unpleasant bodily symptoms—a panic attack. This is the body's way of "keeping score."

## Why Agoraphobics May Withhold Their Feelings

Agoraphobics have a tremendous need to control themselves and their environments yet often feel they will be unable to control how they express feelings, doing so inappropriately. For example, Fannie, a woman who went through recovery the same time I did, was always afraid she would say something ridiculous or embarrassing or act on a destructive or negative emotional impulse.

Other sufferers are afraid they will not be able to control feelings once they express them. As Cara, a New York woman, said, "I'm afraid once I start crying I will cry uncontrollably." Still others, due to their sensitive, easily stimulated personality, inhibit their feelings because they are unable to tolerate strong feelings in themselves or in others.

As children, some agoraphobics were not free to express their natural feelings or impulses. In addition, the level of intensity of their personality may have bothered their parents. So as children they were told to "calm down." Parents may have said, "It's not ladylike to yell" or "Big boys don't cry." This taught that anger and sadness were not acceptable. Wanting to please mom and dad, they then tried to inhibit these emotions. As adults many continued to hold these feelings in.

Pehaps as children their feelings may have also been frequently discounted or ignored: "You're not really mad at mommy." Perhaps one parent was so explosive that as children the agoraphobics suppressed their feelings to protect themselves. Some may have also made a conscious decision to never be like that parent. Unfortunately, when feelings go unacknowledged or unexpressed, the intensity level of the original feeling increases.

## The Importance of Recognizing and Expressing Feelings

Before sufferers can express their feelings they must learn to recognize exactly what those feelings are. Are they resentment, anger, fear, insecurity? Family support team members should also examine *their* true feelings concerning their loved one's disorder.

Here are five ways to help the sufferer and the support person recognize their feelings:

1. Try to identify the emotions you feel at the time they arise. Ask yourself periodically, "What are my emotions right now?" You may think you feel anger when you really feel resentment.

2. Pretend you are watching someone else experience the same emotions, then try to figure out what that person might be feeling.

3. Verbalize your feelings by talking to someone who is understanding, trustworthy, and non-judgmental—someone who will listen without offering opinions—such as a therapist, a support person, or a very good friend.

4. Write your feelings in a journal or dictate them into a tape recorder. To give yourself a good perspective about these feelings and insight into the issues that may be running your life look at them again in a few weeks or months.

5. Write sentences that begin with "I feel angry because . . . ," "I feel depressed because . . . ," "I feel anxious because . . . ," and so forth. If you find you can't finish the sentence, don't worry; the words may come later.

Sufferers should acknowledge what they feel inside, then allow themselves to let the feelings out. If they feel like crying, they should cry. If they are angry, they should constructively vent that anger. They should also learn to tolerate and accept all their feelings, including the bad, without judging whether they are right or wrong.

Their feelings, however, need to be slowly desensitized by the sufferer expressing them a little at a time. Sharing feelings, especially negative emotions like anger and sadness, help dissolve and diminish the intensity of these feelings, and sharing positive feelings helps to strengthen and expand the good feelings.

Very few sufferers recover without recognizing, accepting, and understanding their feelings and learning to release and express them. This is just as important as all the other recovery skills.

## FEELINGS OF ANGER

Because many agoraphobics endured anger and criticism within their families as they grew up, they intensely dislike anger and are afraid of being overwhelmed by it. This often makes them unaware of their own angry feelings and unable to express them constructively. Recognizing this hidden anger can reduce anxiety.

Society often regards angry and aggressive feelings as "bad," thus we have a tendency to deny these feelings or to conceal, restrain, or inhibit them. With an agoraphobic, anger may start as a minor aggravation, but if ignored, it continues to build as other aggravations add to it. If the process continues, minor aggravations combine to become one large powder keg waiting to blow. Often this anger comes out as an illogical, sporadic blast that makes little or no sense to anyone, including the sufferer.

As a Kentucky woman explained, "I would throw a temper tantrum over some little thing, then feel bad because I didn't know why I became so upset."

Family support team members should realize that this "blast" is not only okay but normal. Sometimes at first, it's even necessary. Adult agoraphobics usually have a stock way of expressing negative emotions such as frustration, anger, guilt, shame, or grief. They often hold in their emotions for long periods, afraid that their spouses will leave them if they express their true feelings.

Dr. Hardy expressed it this way: "They may feel their emotions only as vague discomforts, describing them as a physical symptom like an upset stomach or dizziness. And when they can no longer stand the pressure of these unexpressed emotions, they erupt into a rage or a crying jag."

Besides creating a verbal explosion, these angry feelings often cause a variety of ailments such as headaches, insomnia, ulcers, diarrhea, depression, and so on. As a matter of fact, sufferers can become so afraid of releasing their anger and the destruction letting go might cause that it can result in a no-holes-barred #10 panic attack (described in Chapter 1).

To best help your afflicted loved one when he or she erupts in a fit of anger or a crying jag, assure this person that you will not leave and that you still love him or her. Linda from California said, "I can't tell you how helpful it was to have a strong shoulder to cry on any time I needed it, as well as a reliable one to lean on."

Remember that this person is not reacting toward you with angry feelings, but toward a lifetime of self-doubt and criticism. Don't take it as a personal attack. If your loved one becomes angry, this means he or she feels sure enough of your love to take the risk of expressing anger. Have patience. As the sufferer recovers this person will learn new methods of coping with powerful feelings before reaching the boiling point. The feelings will also eventually become more appropriate to the circumstance and easier for you both to understand and cope with.

### Self-Directed Anger

Dr. Hardy found that self-hatred is common among those who suffer from agoraphobia. Agoraphobics may hate themselves not only for their condition, but for being too fearful to live a normal life. They also hate others because of their abilitiy to go places and do things sufferers themselves cannot do.

As Stacy, a California woman, explained, "I find myself looking at people who are happy, or those who are driving a car by themselves, and I resent them."

When self-hatred becomes strong enough, it can lead to self-punishment, which can prevent sufferers from recovering. Some sufferers are so full of self-hatred that they unconsciously behave in ways that are destined to end in failure.

The first step in overcoming this problem is to become aware of it. The next step is to realistically figure out what the negative self-defeating behaviors are, then to examine how each of these behaviors holds back recovery. The final step is to accept, confront, and alter the negative behavior, instead of being moved by it or avoiding it.

Let's start by taking inventory. Here is a checklist of the most common self-defeating behaviors that affect sufferers (many of which are unconscious):

1. *Perfectionism.* Sufferers often set unrealistic goals and standards for themselves and others. Even when they achieve normal or above-normal levels, they may see themselves as failures. Sufferers need to understand they are worthwhile, regardless of their achievements. They also must realize they will have less anxiety and feel better about themselves if they set smaller, more realistic goals.

2. *Exaggeration.* Agoraphobics often exaggerate the bad and underestimate or refuse to accept the good. Often they dwell on a negative thought until it frightens them. They also tend to overlook their good traits and be overly critical of their bad ones. When they receive a compliment, they change it into a criticism. They might say, "If I had taken more time, it could have been better." Sufferers need to be more positive about themselves, their thoughts, and their lives.

3. *Overemphasizing, or giving one's imagination too much power.* Emotionally, sufferers may make routine tasks seem overwhelming, or they may confuse actual fears with imaginary fears. They may also worry about the future, rather than enjoying the present. And they may imagine others are thinking and feeling negative things about them. Sufferers need to realize that making a task seem overwhelming may be an excuse for not trying. They also need to learn how to test their fears and thoughts for reality (discussed in Chapter 10).

4. *Procrastination.* Sufferers often put off solving their problems. They may also misuse alcohol or drugs as a way to avoid facing or solving problems. They may hesitate trying new things because of past failures or hurts. These sufferers need to take an honest look at themselves. Are they self-sabotaging? If so, they should get professional help to overcome this.

5. *Placing blame, complaining, or making excuses.* They may see themselves as agoraphobic to make an excuse for themselves or to have a condition they can blame others for. They may also nit-pick and nag about their lives, the disorder, recovery, and so on, all of which relieve them of having to look to themselves to recover.

They may also label themselves negatively, using the labels as an excuse to relinquish control: "I can't help it; I'm handicapped." Sufferers must realize that they alone are responsible for their own recovery. Others can help, but only the sufferers can perform the recovery steps. They also must realize that negatively labeling will not help recovery.

6. *Refusing to make changes.* Sufferers may hold on to old familiar ways instead of substituting more successful ones. They may also mentally review past hurts, keeping them alive in their emotions. Sufferers need to risk trying new ways. They also need to realize the importance of discussing past hurts with a therapist or trusted friend in order to let go.

7. *Refusing to accept help.* Sufferers may believe that they should be able to recover or work out problems on their own. As a result, they continually refuse outside help. Sufferers need to realize that accepting help is a sign of strength and that helping makes others feel good because they feel needed.

8. *Self-blame.* Sufferers nearly always assume the blame rests on them. Sometimes they take responsibility for every bad event. If the children get bad grades, it's the sufferer's fault. If the spouse drinks, it's the sufferer's fault. If others get angry or cry, it's the sufferer's fault. They may over-blame themselves for every mistake they've ever made. These sufferers need to understand that they can't be blamed for the actions of others. They must also realize that everyone makes mistakes. In reality, they must replace self-blame with the love and compassion they normally give to others.

9. *Giving too much credence to others.* Sufferers often take the words of others as those of an expert. They may also give others the power to make the sufferer's decisions. Or they may continually compare themselves to others, always putting themselves down. Sufferers need to take responsibility for themselves and have faith in their own abilities. They should also realize that comparing themselves to others is a waste of time, for no two people are the same. And they should never compare their recovery to that of other sufferers. Each person recovers at his or her own speed.

.   .   .

## Dealing with Angry Feelings

To keep anger from ending in a powerful burst of emotions, Dr. Hardy found sufferers must learn to *recognize* early warning signals. They must *express* anger the minute it's recognized, and *talk this anger out* reasonably and logically.

Sufferers and support people should try to use anger, rather than lose it. For instance, when either the sufferer or the support person becomes angry at the other, he or she can use that energy to talk about the problem.

When the anger level is high, however, it needs to be discharged first before it can be discussed. Here are some ways to ventilate and release angry feelings. When very angry, exercise vigorously, hit the bed with a toy bat or a rolled-up newspaper, scream into a pillow, pound your fists, hit a punching bag, pull weeds, or chop wood.

Verbally discharge moderate anger by sharing it with a trusted friend who is not associated with the problem. Write out your feelings. Write letters to whoever angered you, expressing your thoughts. When finished, put the letters away for a day or two, then decide whether or not you want to send them—chances are you won't.

Once anger is defused, solve the problem by discussing it with the appropriate people. With less intense anger share your feelings with a confidant first before directly confronting the person that angered you. If slightly angered, confront the situation or count to ten, taking in some slow, deep breaths.

Developing a wide range of assertive skills to replace aggressive behavior is extremely helpful in dealing with anger, especially for the sufferer. (Assertiveness is discussed in Chapter 10.) Here are some ways I learned to deal with anger during recovery:

1. Determine your anger's source. Ask: "Why am I angry?" "What do I really want?" "Do I feel threatened? If so, how?" If you have trouble discovering the source, ask a trusted relative or friend not related to the difficulty to help.

2. Once the source is determined, decide exactly what made you angry. Writing about your anger may help. Also ask yourself,

"Is my anger appropriate to the situation?" Kicking the dog, for example, because you're angry at your spouse is not appropriate.

3. Ask yourself what it would take to make the situation right, thinking about what you really want and need. Then list several constructive suggestions for improving the problem.

4. Rehearse these constructive suggestions. This will help you later to clearly communicate to someone why you are angry and clearly share your suggestions for the situation.

5. Communicate your suggestions and why you are angry to a trusted friend or relative not involved in the problem. Then practice doing so until you feel comfortable enough for an actual confrontation.

6. Confront the real problem and whoever is involved with it. When you feel the anger rising, stop and take a breather, stepping away until the intensity of your emotions lessen.

Expressing anger lets the sufferer take control of the situation. When this person identifies, expresses, and resolves the angry feelings and gets some of his or her wants and needs met, this person will feel better and have fewer areas of anxiety. The intensity of the anger will also rapidly decrease.

Sufferers must learn to not be afraid of their anger and to express their anger where it is warranted, such as standing up for themselves and not letting themselves be put down. They must make an effort to stop their belief that they must please others or be nice in every situation. And both the sufferer and the support person need to learn ways to communicate without blaming, criticizing, or judging.

Your perceptions and thoughts of what is said or done, and the significance you place on them, create your feelings of anger. Nobody can make you angry. And your anger changes only you, not others. As soon as you begin to express your emotions, they start to change.

## FEELINGS OF SEPARATION AND LOSS

Many agoraphobics have suffered from separation anxiety. Feelings of anger, separation, and loss are difficult for sufferers to handle. Due to the agoraphobic's highly emotional personality, these experiences often cause strong reactions. Abandonment, rejection, and intense grief are expressed as withdrawal, sadness, and depression, arousing anxiety and fear in many sufferers.

Agoraphobics often feel a sense of separation, loss, or aloneness even when the individual these feelings relate to is physically present. In addition, anything that lowers self-esteem causes an agoraphobic to feel loss. This includes withdrawal of affection or rejection, such as a boy being chosen last for the baseball team or a girl not being invited to a birthday party. Even an adult who doesn't get a promotion can suffer a form of loss.

In more serious circumstances this includes the death of a loved one, the breakup of a relationship, or a parent's divorce. Even perceived or dreaded losses—losses that haven't happened yet—can cause some people to experience these feelings.

Loss and separation are painful emotions for everyone. But they are especially difficult for sufferers, who are afraid to express emotions. In addition, any person who experiences loss and separation and can't express these feelings can experience a variety of frightening sensations such as detachment, emptiness, disorientation, knots in their stomach, plus physical symptoms like insomnia, stomach cramps, distorted eyesight, and over-tiredness.

Members of the family support team must recognize the need for sufferers to express their feelings. This helps sufferers recover from these emotions and their consequences and shows them that they have the strength to survive and overcome these feelings.

## THE IMPORTANCE OF LOVE

Love is a powerful resource. Dr. Hardy believed this so strongly that he included a lesson on love in the Terrap recovery program. As he said, "Everyone needs love, for it is the most powerful of all the feelings." For the sufferer, the feeling of love helps them to feel safe, secure, and accepted. Love is a critical part of the phobic nest, discussed in Chapter 6.

Unfortunately, many agoraphobics believe that their differences, the qualities that make them unique, will not be tolerated or accepted by others. As a result, in trying to be like others, many grow up conforming to others' beliefs and wishes in order to get approval and to keep from being rejected. But not being who they really want to be makes it difficult for them to love themselves.

Because they have become so self-critical, they often fail to recognize or accept friendship and affection from others. Their inhibition and lack of self-expression also makes it hard for them to express positive emotions or gestures. For example, when someone pays them a compliment or smiles at them, they often feel uncomfortable.

Society's taboos can lessen an agoraphobic's ability to give and receive love—for example, such taboos as "Don't speak to strangers," "Don't touch other people," "Never smile at someone you don't know." These no-no's handicap agoraphobics, for they inhibit their social interaction with others.

In *A Complete Guide to Your Emotions and Your Health,* Emrika Padus and the editors of Prevention Magazine report that when people feel loved the cells in their body create a healthy biological reaction similar to the effects of good diet and fitness. Love, they believe, is a great stress reducer. When sufferers feel love and support from relatives and others, they seem to overcome their ailments better. Unconditional love shown by a spouse is especially helpful.

Dr. Bernard Siegel, author of *Love, Medicine, and Miracles,* says, "I am convinced that unconditional love is the most powerful known stimulant of the immune system. The truth is 'love heals.'" Dr. Siegel stresses the importance of people completely loving themselves, as well as others. No matter what the disorder, he believes chances of recovery are much better when there is self-love along with a strong loving relationship. With these things, you can get through almost anything.

Some experts believe the effects of love are cumulative. Much the same as squirrels store nuts for the winter, people can stockpile good feelings inside their psyches to help them deal with the tough times. Then, when everything in their lives seems bad, their accumulated good feelings act as a perpetual reminder that life is still good, thus making coping with the difficulties much easier.

How can you and other members of the family support team help? You can establish a loving relationship between you and the sufferer and encourage this person to express and share feelings. You can encourage him or her to not be afraid to be him- or herself and to accept being different from others. You can work to share common interests, goals, and activities together with this person. And you can encourage collaboration and a shared concern for one another, along with the togetherness of working as a team. Allow some give and take and accept the sufferer's faults and weaknesses, while keeping criticism to a minimum. Allow the sufferer to develop his or her own identity and encourage physical and emotional affection between you.

Support people must realize how vital their love and affection can be to the sufferer. As Andrea, a California woman, pointed out, "In the beginning, support people are often our only 'link' to the outside world. Therefore, we must completely rely on the love and affection we receive from this link."

### Self-Love

According to therapist/consultant Peter Hansen, "Self-love is simply the most creative use of our own energy." There are many ways for people to channel that energy: by eating good foods, exercising, doing positive things for themselves. People who have self-love treat themselves in a caring way. For sufferers, the energy of self-love can be channeled into performing the recovery techniques. Self-love is also a good way for them to overcome their emotional dependence on others for their value as people.

## LENDING AN EMOTIONAL EAR

You can help the sufferer most simply by being there when your loved one wants to talk about his or her feelings. My interviews show how important it is for you to be there emotionally. Jillian, a California woman, said, "The best thing my support person did was to let me talk about my feelings and fears at the moment I needed to and truly listen, listen, listen." Jane, a woman from Virginia, said, "Listening quietly and letting me run the gamut of my feelings, then helping me to sort them out by allowing me to freely and openly discuss them without criticizing, was a tremendous help." And Peter, a man from Ohio, happily explained, "Just listening to me verbalize my emotional problems was one of the best things my support person did to help me get well."

# Let's Talk: Good Communication and Negotiation Recovery Skills

*"To think justly, we must understand what others mean; to know the value of our thoughts, we must try their effect on other minds."*

*—William Hazlitt, The Plain Speaker*

## COMMUNICATION

Before walking the steps towards recovery, you, the other support people, and the sufferer must learn to communicate effectively.

The purpose of communication during the recovery process is to enable the sufferer and the support team to understand what each does and doesn't want and what each thinks and feels. All support members must be able to openly discuss their agreements and disagreements. Good communication skills will reduce the amount of frustration and stress the support team and the sufferer must endure because of the ailment.

As Kyle, one California husband, says, "I can't stress enough the need to open up lines of communication so that anxieties the sufferer encounters have a way of being released. Learning to communicate better while working the recovery steps together gave us fertile grounds for exploring our relationship. It also opened up topics to discuss we would not have otherwise touched on."

Before we take a look at communication techniques, you and the sufferer first need to evaluate how well your present relationship functions. Ask yourself these questions:

Do we have a strong commitment to the relationship? Does the relationship come before my or the sufferer's self-interests? Do both of us give as well as get something out of the relationship? Do we share a strong working alliance? Are we working together on recovery? Do we work to maintain and improve the relationship? Do we share common recovery goals? Do we plan ways to approach and achieve these goals *together*? Do I give the sufferer the same love, honesty, respect, attention, and openness that I expect to receive in return?

Answering no to any of these questions signals a problem that needs to be addressed. Supported recovery is a team effort. When only one person is willing to make the necessary changes, recovery becomes extremely difficult.

While most of the time you will be in a partnership, there are times you or other members of the support team will have individual problems growing out of the recovery process that need to be addressed. Stan, for example, was overly impatient and realized he needed to work on being a better support person. He discussed this with his wife Betty, letting her know he couldn't change his ingrained behavior overnight, but he would do his best to subdue it. While his impatience when practicing facing her fears had been a problem for Betty, she respected the fact that he needed time to handle the problem.

Communicating about one another's problems will help you grow individually through recovery while still growing closer as a team. There must always be full communication with no one-sided decisions. A consolidated front doubles your resources affords a much stronger position from which to approach problems.

The following communication techniques offer both the sufferer and the support team guidelines to use during recovery.

.    .    .

## The Three Categories of Communication

Dr. Hardy put communication into the following three categories:

*Self-communication* is what we say to ourselves. It can be *verbal*, as when we talk out loud, or *non-verbal,* as expressed by our thinking or internal dialogue. Self-talk helps us make decisions and judgments and set goals. Self-talk is an important part of the sufferer's recovery.

*Communication with others* also can be verbal and non-verbal. Verbal communication falls into four categories: feelings, observations, thoughts, and needs. Each category requires different styles of expression and usually a different vocabulary. Non-verbal dialogue uses body messages such as a grin or a grimace, a certain look, a particular posture, or a shrug of the shoulders. Non-verbal messages aren't always clear, but they provide clues to what the other person needs.

*Non-communication* is known as "small talk," such as, "How are you today?" Most of the time the person asking doesn't want an answer or care how the other person thinks or feels, for he or she is just being polite.

To communicate means to interchange, share, or make known thoughts, feelings, and information and to connect with another. Thus, communication can not only create or maintain a relationship, it can destroy one as well. Communication can also be a thermometer for monitoring the temperature of a relationship.

While not everyone communicates well, all people communicate at some level. People cannot *not* communicate, for even silence says something. However, the problem some people have in their communication is that they fail to connect with one another. This is often the plight of sufferers and their support people.

## Forms of Expression

Let's take a look at the four kinds of expression that people use to communicate with one another, as adapted from the book *Messages* by McKay, Davis, and Fanning:

*Observations* report what your senses tell you. They are formed by what you have heard, read, or personally experienced. For example, "I heard on the news that it's going to be hot tomorrow," "I read about the accident in the newspaper," or "I had a flat tire this morning."

*Thoughts* are based on the conclusions drawn from what you have read, observed, or heard. They may embody right or wrong judgments which lead to beliefs and opinions—for example, an opinion such as "Butter tastes better than margarine," a belief such as "Honesty is essential for a good relationship," or a judgement such as "You were wrong to talk to him that way."

*Feelings* are your emotions and sensibility. When others know what you are feeling, they often have more understanding and empathy for you. It also puts them in a better position to meet your needs. Feeling statements might be "I feel anxious when left alone," "I feel angry when you talk to me that way," or "When I finally got my raise, I was elated."

*Needs* are declarations about what would help or please you. They are not judgmental or place blame. It is impossible to have a close relationship when needs are not expressed. When people clearly state their needs to one another, their relationship grows and changes. Examples of need statements are "I'm exhausted; can you feed the dogs tonight?" "Could you be home by seven? We're having friends for dinner," or "Would you just hold my hand?"

## Using Whole Messages

All four expressions used simultaneously are called *whole messages*. Relationships are enriched when whole messages are used. To maintain a thriving relationship with partners, relatives, and close friends you must share all your experiences—what you think, feel, observe, and need. Let them know what you see and what your conclusions are. Explain how that makes you feel. If you see potential to change a situation, or if you need something, ask or make a suggestion.

John's wife wanted to get well. Since he was willing to devote his time to help her recover, he found her lack of desire to practice confusing and upsetting. When he tried to encourage her to practice, he said, "She felt my encouragement was an attempt to control her." Finally, he explained to her that what he *observed* was her doing nothing. Therefore, he *thought* she wasn't putting forth any effort, and that made him *feel* angry since he was willing to devote the time. He said he still wanted to help, but that he *needed* her to try more. She admitted that facing her fears was so uncomfortable she put it off. "Once I communicated what was going on with me and she explained how she felt, we worked things out together."

To keep your relationship healthy during and after recovery, you must not mask your anger or withhold your needs and wants from one another or other members of the support team. Not using whole messages—sharing only part of what you see, think, feel or need—often leaves others confused and distrustful. No one can understand your anger if you don't let them know why you are angry or frustrated or let them understand your needs when they're not expressed.

This list of four questions from *Messages* will test whether your messages are whole or partial.

1. Have I expressed what I actually know to be fact? Is it based on what I've observed, read, or heard?

2. Have I expressed and clearly labeled my inferences and conclusions?

3. Have I expressed my feelings without blame or judgement?

4. Have I shared my needs without blame or judgement?

To give whole messages you must examine your own internal experiences. Be aware of what it is you are feeling, thinking, observing, and needing. What is the reason for the communication? What is the message you need to get across? Recognizing and using whole messages may take some practice. So go over things in your mind until the messages you want to convey are clear. If need be, work them out on paper.

When you have an essential issue to discuss, first find the proper environment in which to talk. This environment should be a quiet place that is non-distracting and private. It should also be one that is physically comfortable and compatible for both of you.

Before you deliver any message of importance, consider

whether the other person is calm or anxious, cheerful or angry. Is the timing convenient or will this person be hurried?

When communicating, become aware of whether or not your message is getting across. How is the listener responding? Watch the person's facial expressions and body language. Pay attention to eye contact. Is he or she asking questions? Are you getting feedback?

## Keeping Communication Open and Honest

Honesty and openness must be a top priority when making a commitment to communication.

Often patterns of communication taught by parents act as roadblocks to being open and honest. These roadblocks consist of *don't talk* rules such as "Don't talk about your feelings," "Don't tell about Dad's alcoholism [or some other family secret]," "Don't disagree or show anger," "Don't talk about sex," "Don't admit your mistakes," and so on. The result often is unexpressed feelings that cause tension to build.

Listen to yourself and your loved one to discover which *don't talk* rules each of you now lives by. Unspoken conflicts can develop from mismatched rules. Because we live by one rule, we sometimes expect others to do the same. Yet they may be living by another rule. Discuss differences, because free exchange of all feelings—positive and negative—develops closeness.

## Guidelines for Good Communication

These guidelines will help improve communication skills:

*Establish open communication* by being as honest as possible about your thoughts and feelings with other people. Open and honest feedback brings openness and honesty in return. The more people you openly communicate with, the more you open up the avenues for feedback and help. Honesty, however, is no excuse for harming someone. Some types of honesty can inhibit relationships rather than promote them.

*Think before speaking.* Use consideration. Make sure you are clear about what you think, feel, and want before you talk. This helps communicate the message clearly and effectively.

*Use "I" statements, and avoid "You" statements.* "I" statements allow you to express your feelings without placing blame or causing the other person to become defensive. For instance, instead of saying, "You are very insulting," say, "I felt like that was an insult; it hurt me." "You" statements are accusatory and often lead to a win-lose argument rather than to honest communication. Be careful not to say, "I think that you . . ." or "I feel that you. . . ." These are only "you" statements in disguise. Try saying, "I want . . . " or "I don't want . . . ," "I feel . . . " or "I don't feel . . . ," leaving the word *you* out all together.

*Be positive, specific, and remain focused* when expressing your thoughts, feelings, and wants. First, point out to your partner what you like about him or her. Then rephrase what you don't like in positive terms. Instead of saying, "Don't be so demanding," say, "I like it so much better when you ask me rather than tell me." In lieu of saying, "I wish you would be more thoughtful," say, "I would really appreciate it if you would call when you're going to be late." Let the person know exactly what you think, feel, or want, and remain focused by keeping your goal in mind. If other topics wander into the conversation, come back to the original subject.

*Actively listen and observe.* Concentrate on what the other person is saying. Watch body language and demeanor and listen to tone of voice. Ask the other person to share his or her thoughts and feelings. Ask that individual to paraphrase what he or she thinks you said. If you were misinterpreted, correct it.

*Don't force communication.* The right time for you may be the wrong time for the other person. Ask first if the time is right, then respect the other person's wishes, scheduling for another time if necessary. However, when it is an issue that is essential to your relationship, make it as soon as possible.

*Set limits as to what is allowed during communication.* Discussions should never be allowed to cross the line of mutual respect. When discussions become abusive or unhealthy, they are no longer productive. You have several choices. You can simply make no comment. You can say, "It's too bad to feel that way." Or if it is especially objectionable, you can say, "I will no longer listen to this, as I find your behavior unacceptable."

*Thank the person for communicating with you.* When you positively reinforce others by thanking them, they are more likely to be receptive in the future. Don't expect communication to be perfect. However, when you follow the communication guidelines, even when you don't succeed, you still improve your ability to communicate. The more you use these skills, the more they develop.

## Message Filters

Dr. Hardy said that when a message is sent it must filter through *feelings*, for every word that the speaker says is influenced by his or her feelings. He said the message must also filter through *beliefs*, because the speaker's words are influenced by his or her set beliefs—opinions, judgments, and expectations. The message must also filter through *logic* to enable the message to follow an appropriate course of reasoning.

The person's feelings, set beliefs, and logic influence the way the message is given, as well as the way it is received. When feelings get stronger, logic gets weaker and beliefs render more influence. But when both people learn how to properly communicate, it lessens the complications derived from the filters.

# ACTIVE LISTENING

Active listening skills are essential to maintaining good relationships. Sufferers say that one of the things they look for most in support people is the ability to listen. As one California man said, "The feeling that I could talk to my support person and know she would always listen was valuable, beyond measure."

Listening shows you care. A good listener can put aside his or her own set beliefs, prejudices, and self-interest. This enables the listener to understand the other persons feelings, and see things through the other person's perspective.

Listening does not mean saying nothing. Listening requires participation. In order to understand what is being communicated, you need to ask questions and respond with feedback. The dialogue becomes part of the communication process.

## Guidelines for Active Listening

· To avoid misunderstanding, paraphrase back to the speaker what you think he or she said. Here are some sample lead-ins; "What I heard you say was . . . ," "To my understanding, what was happening was . . . ," "What you mean is . . . ," or "In other words, you said. . . ."

· Ask questions. Request more information and background on what's being said, but don't interrupt. Questioning helps clarify the speaker's message. Maintain good eye contact, and lean forward slightly to show interest.

· Give the speaker feedback by expressing your feelings, thoughts, and perceptions about what was said. This should be done without stating approval or disapproval and without passing judgment. Feedback is a good method to see if what you perceived from the communication was correct. Feedback should be given immediately; the longer you wait the less valuable it becomes.

· Be objective. Do not let your feelings, beliefs, or logic contaminate the message. Try to hear the entire message before placing judgment. To do this, pretend you are the other person. Try to see things from his or her point of view.

· Listen with awareness and observe the speaker as a whole. Listen to the words and tone of voice. Watch the person's facial expressions, gestures, body language, and posture. Do they fit the message's content? If not, clarify the discrepancy through feedback. Use both your head and your gut feelings to determine what the other person is saying.

## Blocks to Being a Good Listener

Listening blocks often get in the way of effective communication. Here are the most common listening blocks, as adapted from the book *Messages*.

· Comparing yourself to the speaker. This makes it difficult to listen because you're thoughts are continually trying to determine which of you is smarter, more emotionally stable, who has suffered the most, and so on.

· Being a mind reader, trying to figure out what the speaker is feeling and thinking. You distrust what is said, so instead of paying attention to the words, you go by your intuition, your hunches, and your speculations.

· Rehearsing future comments. You try to look interested, but your attention is focused solely on preparing what you'll say. This often keeps you from hearing what is being said.

· Filtering part of the words out; listening to some, but not all. You listen just enough to find out if the speaker is sad or angry, for example. If everything is okay, your mind wanders and you stop listening. You may avoid or not remember hearing anything that's perceived as critical, unpleasant, or threatening.

· Judging the speaker. You place negative labels on the speaker and stop paying attention to what he or she says. You may judge a person's statements as crazy, immoral, stupid, and so on.

· Dreaming. Your mind drifts off to something else, sometimes due to something said that triggers memories, and you get only part of the speaker's message. It can indicate lack of interest in this person or lack of commitment on your part.

· Identifying what the speaker says with your personal experiences. It reminds you of something you've felt or done. You may even jump in with your statement before the speaker is finished.

· Advising the speaker. You don't acknowledge his or her message, or you miss how this person really feels and immediately plunge in with advice.

· Sparring with the speaker. You are quick to disagree, argue, or debate. You may dismiss the speaker's viewpoint by being sarcastic, or you may discount what this person says.

· Being right is so important, you will do anything to avoid being wrong. You'll accuse, twist facts, make excuses, shout, and refuse to take criticism or advice.

· Derailing the conversation by changing the subject when it makes you uncomfortable or bored. To avoid listening, you may joke everything off, responding to what is said in jest.

· Placating. You are pleasant, friendly, and supportive because you want the speaker to like you, but you don't want to be involved. Your replies mean nothing.

·    ·    ·

# NEGOTIATION AND COMPROMISE

Maintaining a good relationship requires negotiation and compromise. Learning to negotiate and compromise will help both the sufferer and the support person get what they want without alienating one another.

Often agoraphobics do not have their wants and needs satisfied, partly from lack of negotiation skills and partly because they fail to make their needs known. Sometimes even when they are able to express their needs it is in the form of demands. When their needs go unfulfilled, sufferers angrily protest or withdraw into their shell. Dr. Hardy called this "either/or, all-or-nothing" behavior.

To counter this, sufferers need to learn to negotiate their wants and needs. Support people must also learn to negotiate. Negotiation brings both to an equal position, helping them to resolve conflicts to one another's mutual satisfaction.

## Guidelines for Good Negotiation and Compromise

Negotiation and compromise take honest communication, a dedication to the same goal, and combined commitment to solve the problem. Both people must agree to do whatever they can to change themselves, the situation, or both.

Here are some general guidelines:

1. Be aware that a problem exists, obtain a clear idea of what that problem is, and be willing to negotiate and compromise.

2. Consider what each of you is seeing, hearing, and feeling and what you both want. Observe all the clues.

3. Select a time to get together and a place that is mutually agreeable. Timing is important; participants should be well rested, relaxed, in a good mood, and not preoccupied with other things. Choose comfortable seating opposite one another (not too close or far away) and without barriers between you.

4. Share your findings. Acknowledge the other person's perceptions, but have enough persistence and self-confidence to get your message across.

5. Pinpoint and discuss what you both hope to accomplish, setting some goals and priorities. If necessary, write these down.

6. Take responsibility individually and as a team to provide actions or solutions that help reconcile the problem to both your satisfactions.

7. Discuss the positive and negative aspects of each solution or action. Employ give-and-take if needed. Be willing to compromise your less important priorities to meet the other person's more important ones.

8. Decide on a plan of action, then commit to it as a team. Finally, agree to a trial period for a set duration.

9. After a period of time, decide what has and has not worked. If one of you is not satisfied with the outcome, try an alternate solution or action following the same procedure of negotiation and compromise.

10. Thank those involved for cooperating. This will smooth the way for and benefit future negotiations.

## What Interferes with Negotiation and Compromise

Dr. Hardy stressed that certain thoughts, experiences, and actions interfere with negotiation and compromise.

1. Negative past experiences that bring back memories and stir up feelings. Postpone negotiations and take time to discuss these past events before proceeding.

2. Ultimatums that turn the negotiation process into a two-choice situation of being either/or, all-or-nothing. This negates all negotiation and compromise.

3. Overstating the issue. Once your point is made, be quiet and give the other person a chance to respond.

4. Saying no. This brings negotiation and compromise to a complete halt. Ask if, given more facts, the "no" is open to further discussion. If possible, delay a final decision until the individual reconsiders the facts or until you receive more information.

5. Subjective thinking based on feelings or temperament instead of the facts. This interferes with negotiation and compromise. Everyone's feelings must conform to the reality of the situation.

6. Being too hard-nosed or letting personal principles stand in the way. To counter this, politely ask the other person to explain or back up these principles. Listen for errors in logical thinking. If necessary, discontinue negotiations until the problem is worked out or the principles can be fully explored.

These rules of good communication and the negotiation and compromise guidelines will help you, the sufferer, and the entire team make decisions and solve problems in a positive way.

# Roadside Service for a Successful Journey

*"The means prepare the end, and the*
*end is what the means have made it."*

*—John Morley, Critical Miscellanies*

There are some other basic techniques the sufferer will need to apply on the road to recovery. They include learning assertiveness skills and positive visualization; overcoming negative self-talk, cognitive distortions, and false beliefs; using countering, affirmations, and reality testing; and stopping destructive thoughts. Many recovery programs utilize these or silimar techniques.

## ASSERTIVENESS SKILLS

To learn to express feelings, wants, and needs sufferers must learn to be more assertive. Being assertive is a way for sufferers to be honest with themselves as well as with others. It also reduces the sufferer's anxiety level.

Since sufferers feel the need to please everyone, they are generally non-assertive or passive. Unfortunately, this behavior only spawns more anxiety. To learn to be assertive the sufferer must first learn to differentiate between passive, aggressive, and assertive behavior.

*Passive behavior* is not directly expressing feelings, wants, and needs. Passive people generally say yes or make excuses rather than saying no. They find it hard to make requests or give opinions.

*Aggressive behavior* (often confused with assertive behavior) concerns being on the attack and trying to control or dominate other people.

*Assertive behavior* is directly expressing one's feelings, wants and needs to other people while respecting their feelings, wants, and needs in return.

Instead of being openly aggressive, some people tend to be passive-aggressive. They express anger or aggressive feelings in a roundabout way by being passively resistant. They may whine or complain, or they may, for example, be late for something they didn't want to attend in the first place.

The primary elements of assertive messages are . . .

. . . clearly knowing what you want. Some people think they want one thing when they really want another. For example, a wife may complain to a spouse about him watching too much football, when all she really wants is more attention.

. . . knowing how to ask for what you want using direct language that clearly explains how you feel.

. . . suggesting the outcome you would like the message to accomplish. Use "I" messages, rather than "you" messages.

While not easy, allowing the sufferer to express him- or herself assertively has many benefits. It lessens the person's anxiety, leads to gained confidence and self-esteem, and increases willingness to attempt more things and take more risks.

## SELF-TALK

Our internal self-talk determines our frame of mind. It affects our feelings, moods, thoughts, attitudes, and behavior; thus it influences our judgments and decisions. If we internally say, "Why did I get myself into this situation? I can't handle this, I've got to leave," the entire reaction is one of fear, anxiety, and frustration.

Self-talk can tell sufferers that a situation is dangerous before anything frightening happens, and it occurs so subtly it seems as if the situation made them afraid. Their scary self-talk maintains sufferers' fearful avoidance, and avoidance maintains scary thinking and self-talk, creating a vicious cycle.

Sufferers must change this negative inner dialogue into positive self-talk that will give them more helpful and realistic feedback. They must also continually pay attention to what they say to themselves. "Instead of popping a pill," as one recovering agoraphobic explained, "I now use relaxation and self-talk, telling myself things like 'You're not going to die; relax and the fear will subside.'"

Another technique I found beneficial is to mentally say, "Stop," picturing a big red stop sign. When repeated enough, this enables a person to disrupt negative thinking on the spot, turning it off like a light switch.

# WHAT-IF THINKING

"What-if" thinking, mentioned earlier, is a part of the sufferers' negative, fear inducing self-talk. For instance, they say, "What if I have a panic attack in the store?" or "What if my car breaks down and I can't get home?" If they ask themselves enough "what-if's," they avoid the situation all together and worsen their fear and anxiety.

To recover, sufferers must replace the what-if's with positive, rational statements such as "So what. I'm able to handle this. These are only thoughts, not fact."

The first step in countering the what-if's is to become aware of them. You can help by pointing out when the sufferer is what-if-ing, then suggesting that he or she consciously bring another thought to mind. Suggest counting backwards from one hundred by threes, counting letters on a sign, or repeating positive, encouraging phrases.

Also help the sufferer separate the realistic from the unrealistic. Ask questions such as "Are you out of control?" "Have you passed out?" "Is anyone really watching you?" or whatever else the sufferer believes may happen.

# COGNITIVE DISTORTIONS

Unrealistic, illogical, or distorted thinking, known as cognitive distortions, cause and maintain much of the sufferers' anxiety, depression, self-criticism, and guilt.

When sufferers believe these mental distortions to be true, they make poor judgments. Sufferers must recognize these harmful ways of thinking—a process referred to as cognitive awareness—and counter these thoughts using more realistic and positive self-talk, a process referred to as cognitive restructuring. Here are the ten most common cognitive distortions Dr. Hardy found that sufferers have.

1. *All-or-Nothing, Either/Or Thinking.* Sufferers see things as either right or wrong, black or white, with nothing in between.

2. *Over-Generalization.* Over-generalizers take one incident or bit of evidence and come to a general conclusion.

3. *Labeling.* Over-generalization done in excess.

4. *Mental Filters.* Focusing on negatives and ignoring positives.

5. *Disqualifying the Positive.* Rejecting positive experiences, counting only the negative ones. Dr. Hardy called this the "yeah . . . buts."

6. *Jumping to Conclusions.* Interpreting without evidence, which stems from predicting things from one's own experience or from misreading other people's minds.

7. *Magnification and Catastrophizing (sometimes also called Minimizing).* Erroneously makes every little event into a catastrophe or exaggerates errors, along with a problem's importance.

8. *Emotional Reasoning.* Makes irrational judgments or conclusions based totally on feelings, suspended of all logic.

9. *"Should" Statements.* Having a list of ironclad rules —should's, must's, have-to's, and can't-do's—about how they and others should behave, often stemming from taboos set by others throughout their lives.

10. *Personalization.* Taking everything personally, believing everything said is directed at them. Also inappropriately feeling responsible for almost every occurrence.

These kinds of thinking result in a number of problems. A sufferer will generalize that if they have a panic attack in one grocery store they will have a panic attack in all grocery stores, or if they can barely drive to a grocery store today they will not be able to drive there tomorrow, or they conclude that if they feel helpless, they are helpless. Much of this behavior has been ingrained over a lifetime and will take time and hard work to overcome. Support people can help the sufferer with poor behavior patterns by helping this person reexamine his or her original thinking and by pointing out the truth of the situation.

## FALSE BELIEFS

Sufferers have developed many false or irrational beliefs over their lifetime which they need to overcome in order to recover. Dr. Hardy called these "fallacious beliefs." When sufferers make decisions based on these beliefs without checking them for validity, these beliefs can lead them to make wrong conclusions, resulting in anxiety and other problems such as negative self-talk and cognitive distortions.

The sufferers' present attitude is derived from their erroneous beliefs. When sufferers learn to recognize and dispute these false beliefs and establish new ones that correspond more with reality, it changes their attitude and they begin to take charge of their lives. Since overcoming false beliefs also helps them take control of situations over which they believed they had no control, it also decreases their anxiety.

Following here are a few of the most common mistaken beliefs sufferers have, accompanied by positive counterstatements. These statements are called positive affirmations, and they play a big part in helping to reduce false beliefs and negative self-talk.

*I have to be perfect to be a worthwhile person.*
My self-worth comes from within. Being human, being myself, makes me a worthwhile person.

*If people really knew me, they wouldn't like me.*
What I think of myself is more important than what others think of me. Nobody likes everyone; it's just a fact of life.

*I am powerless over my disorder.*
I am responsible for my own recovery, and I am taking control of my life. Instead of wasting energy convincing myself it is impossible, I am using that energy to accomplish recovery.

*I'm not smart enough, pretty enough, strong enough . . .*
I am a good, valuable person. I believe in myself and will focus on my potential rather than on my limitations.

*I am a victim of my circumstances and therefore have no control over my anxiety.*
The source for an anxious free life lies within me, rather than outside of me. By taking responsibility for my own life, I am making a profound change in the way I approach everything.

As it was with negative self-talk and cognitive distortions, recognizing false beliefs is the first step in overcoming them. The next step for this person is to use positive affirmations to counter negative ones, repeating these counterstatements enough times to implant them into his or her mind. This also works extremely well for countering negative self-talk.

# AFFIRMATIONS

An affirmation is a positive statement that people repeat to themselves about themselves. It is a positive desire for the future, stated in the present tense, as if the desired outcome had already been accomplished. The mind can't tell the difference between what's real and what's not; like a computer it believes whatever is programmed into it and accepts it as fact. By repeatedly telling ourselves we can do something—as in saying, "I *am* calm and relaxed," as opposed to "I *can be* calm and relaxed"—the mind comes to believe it.

You plant a positive "as if" seed, and eventually it germinates and sprouts positive results. Positive affirmations are best if they are short, simple, and very specific. They should also be void of negative words. Instead of a sufferer saying, "I am *not* anxious," which negatively reinforces being anxious, he or she would say, "I am free from anxiety." While the sufferer may feel just the opposite, or may not believe what is being said, by this person repeating the message his or her brain still receives the message and will begin sending it out to his or her body.

Since feelings of phobic anxiety and fear are derived from the subconscious part of the brain feeding such feelings to the conscious part of the brain, affirmations work by reeducating the subconscious to respond to a stimulus in a better way.

The sufferer should begin by making a list of positive affirmations relating to the changes he or she wants to make in his or her life. Then he or she should pick the one that is currently the most important and write that affirmation on a sheet of paper a minimum of fifteen times twice daily for the next three weeks—preferably upon rising and before going to bed. This person should also imagine what he or she will look and sound like when the affirmation is reached. After repeatedly writing an affirmation for just a few days, sufferers will begin to memorize it and can use it anytime and anywhere throughout the day, especially when feeling anxious or low to block out negative self-talk. According to recent studies, it takes twenty-one days to form a new habit. If even a single day is missed, the person must start counting days all over again.

The sufferer can also record a list of affirmations on tape and listen to them while going to sleep, doing chores, or driving. He or she can write them on index cards and tape them various places—on their mirror, the telephone, the TV, above the stove, or, for privacy, in a medicine cabinet or billfold. No matter what method is used, change the affirmations about every three weeks. And remember, daily repetition is the key to success.

## REALITY TESTING AND THE
## IMPORTANCE OF CONTROL

Many sufferers exaggerate the importance of things around them, even small details such as what outfit to wear, what brand of soap to buy, and so on. To overcome this sufferers need to learn to distinguish whether something is important. This is what Dr. Hardy called "reality testing." The support person needs to help the sufferer determine what is and what is not important. This is very beneficial when supporting in-vivo desensitization.

## The Importance of Control

Many sufferers have an intense need to control everything in their environment. This stems from their need to protect themselves from their anxiety and from being surprised by an anxiety attack. However, the need for control renders them uptight and anxious much of the time. Since there are so many things in the world that we have no control over, trying to be in total control of the environment is doomed to failure. For example, people cannot control traffic signals that turn red, buses arriving on time, or the weather. They also cannot control other people's behavior or sometimes how they themselves feel.

Sufferers must learn to control their attitude toward the things they cannot change. For example, if I'm driving on the freeway and the traffic comes to a halt due to an accident ahead, I could become extremely upset. If, instead, I looked at the situation realistically, I would say to myself, "Is there anything I can do about this?" Of course the reality is "no." I can't make the traffic move. And I can't move my car until the accident is cleared away. Since nothing can be done to change the situation, I might as well sit back and relax.

To help the sufferer test the reality of a situation and whether it is worth getting upset over, support people can ask such questions as, "Is there anything you can change about the situation?" If the answer is no, the support person can suggest, "Since you can't do anything about it, have you considered trying to change your attitude toward the situation, so you can at least have some control over how the situation affects you?"

While this is using logic on a disorder that is emotional in nature, this will at least help the sufferer learn to take control of what it is he or she can control. And it will help this person to accept the realities of life and to start making decisions based on them, rather than dwelling on how he or she would like the world to be.

In the beginning, it is important for you and other support

people to relinquish control of all situations involving the sufferer—where they go, how long they stay, which route they take, and so on—to the sufferer. When sufferers are in total control they have less trouble with their anxiety. Any arguing or pressure from you (or others) can instantly bring about the sufferer's anxiety, immediately lessening chances for progress. Once the sufferer's fears have lessened, his or her need to control everything will also decrease, eventually disappearing with the disorder.

## STOPPING DISTURBING THOUGHTS

So often when sufferers are anxious, worried, upset, or anticipating an anxiety-provoking situation, stubborn or frightening thoughts pop into their conscious mind and stay. Often sufferers feel they may have to act on some of these thoughts, which are usually negative and thus could lead to negative results. Hence, these thoughts perpetuate the sufferer's anxiety. While you cannot stop such thoughts, you can help by reminding sufferers of the following techniques. This is especially beneficial when you are helping them practice facing their fears.

In your mind, shout to yourself, "Stop." Then immediately think about something else that is pleasant and nonthreatening, such as a song on the radio, the clouds in the sky, a wonderful vacation, a happy or humorous moment from the past, the color of the room—anything that works. You could also move around, count the change in your pocket, doing some minor physical activity. When unwanted thoughts return, repeat the same thought-stopping process over and over again until successful.

When continually used, this process eventually becomes a habit, making it easier and easier for sufferers to dismiss unwanted thoughts. Sufferers need to stop monitoring their thoughts. They need to learn, too, that they do not have to act on negative thoughts. This involves accepting the fact that it is just a thought, not necessarily a reality. And not worrying about why they had the thought.

.   .   .

# THE MAGIC OF POSITIVE VISUALIZATION

Since merely thinking of a situation can make sufferers feel extremely uncomfortable, positive visualization gives sufferers the chance to imagine or think about a future situation as they would like it to be. When thinking about a future event, such as an in-vivo practice session, an upcoming trip, and so on, instead of imagining having a bad, anxiety-provoking experience, they imagine themselves feeling totally calm, comfortable, and secure in the situation. Sufferers see themselves as confident and able to successfully use the recovery skills.

For example, if it is a trip to the grocery store, sufferers can picture every detail of the store, seeing themselves calmly walking up and down the aisles with the shopping cart. Maybe they see themselves smiling and talking to other people. They see themselves calmly standing in the check-out line and purchasing their groceries. If, while imagining this, they become anxious, they should discontinue the image and use their relaxation skills. When calm, they should return to their positive visualization. With repeated daily use (twenty minutes per time) eventually sufferers will feel no anxiety when thinking about the particular situation. How long it takes for this to occur depends upon the difficulty of the event. Persistence pays off, however, the end result being a significant reduction in anxiety in the real-life situation.

Sufferers can also visualize themselves as they want to be, seeing themselves as having dropped their old destructive patterns and leading dynamic, exciting, anxiety-free lives.

I used the visualization process frequently, especially when taking on new ventures such as my first airplane trip. I practiced this process two or three times a day at first, then slowly progressed to once a day for a month or so before my actual flight. It still amazes me how well it works.

# HELPING SUFFERERS PREPARE
# FOR EXPOSURE PRACTICE

Along with these techniques, the sufferer will also learn the other techniques mentioned in Chapter 3, such as relaxation skills and imaginal and visual desensitization skills. All this will help when he or she begins to do in-vivo desensitization.

Support people can help the sufferer make time alone to practice these techniques. Plan a certain time each day to watch the children, answer the telephone, and make sure there is peace and quiet around the house so the sufferer can practice these skills until he or she becomes proficient.

Before the sufferer can practice facing his or her fears in real life, he or she must have some skills to help him or her do so. This is *vital*. These recovery skills will make the exposure sessions easier on both the sufferer and you, and they will ensure the sufferer eventual success.

Providing the sufferer some time alone for learning recovery skills may seem an inconvenience at the time; however, it will not be forever, and the goal will be well worth the effort for all involved.

## PAVING THE ROAD TO RECOVERY

In addition to the techniques already covered, regular exercise, a well-balanced diet, and a good sense of humor also help pave the road to recovery.

### Physical Exercise

A regular, energetic exercise program releases the sufferers' tension and reduces generalized anxiety. It also helps some sufferers overcome or be less susceptible to their hereditary/biochemical predisposition to panic attacks. It can reduce the severity of panic attacks and lessen the tendency to experience anticipatory anxiety. Studies show exercise also has a substantial antidepressant effect.

Exercise initially creates a physical response similar to anxiety symptoms—thus some sufferers are afraid to exercise—regular exercise over time slows down the heart rate and helps the sufferer stay calmer and have more control over emotions and anxiety. For sufferers who are afraid to exercise, the desensitization process can be used to gradually overcome the frightening feelings experienced when exercising.

Aerobic dancing, brisk walking, running, bicycling, jumping rope, and other aerobic exercises are recommended to reduce general anxiety and the vulnerability to panic attacks. Some researchers believe that forty-five to sixty minutes of moderate exercise like gardening, leisure walking, household chores, or bowling also offer aerobic benefits.

Exercising with an afflicted partner provides support, encouragement, companionship, and motivation. My husband and I took walks, played tennis, and even did yard work together.

Here are some basic tips for starting an exercise program.

· Consult your doctor first.
· Fit workouts into your existing schedule.
· Chose low-impact over high-impact aerobics.
· Set realistic goals.
· Add variety.
· Warm up first.
· Exercise at the optimal level of intensity for your heart.
· Wear suitable footwear and clothing.
· Set a trial period by making a commitment for a specific period of time.
· Maintain an exercise record.

### Good Nutritional Habits

Good nutritional habits and a balanced diet aid anxiety disorder recovery and build stress and anxiety tolerance. Dr. Hardy believed sufferers should eat frequent small meals low in sugar and high in protein and should keep caloric intake in proportion to their weight.

Here are the dietary guidelines for low stress and anxiety reduction (this can benefit support people as well):

· Eliminate stimulants and stress-inducing substances, including caffeine, nicotine, and alcohol.
· Reduce or eliminate simple sugars, replacing them with complex sugars.

- Use salt and sodium products sparingly.
- Reduce intake of foods with cholesterol and animal fats.
- Drink six eight-ounce glasses of water a day.
- Increase intake of dietary fiber.
- Reduce or eliminate allergic foods.
- Maintain a well-balanced, diverse diet following the four basic food groups.
- Use dietary supplements.

## Humor and the Recovery Process

A good sense of humor can be a great ally when working to overcome agoraphobia and panic disorder. Both sufferers and those closely associated with them report that humor was beneficial during the recovery process.

Experts say laughter causes the skeletal muscles to deeply relax and the pulse rate to drop below normal, creating a calming effect. It can also decrease painful conditions—such as headaches, neck aches, and backaches—related to tense muscles caused by anxiety. It also has psychological benefits. According to Norman Cousins, bestselling author of *Anatomy of an Illness,* "Laughter has therapeutic value because it serves as a bulletproof vest that protects you against the ravages of negative emotions."

Many hospitals stress humor and offer patients everything from Play-Doh to comedy videos. A few nursing schools even incorporate "Humor and Health" into their curriculum. Psychologist Frank Prerost of Western Illinois University found that in humor therapy, his patients went through what he calls the "three stages of humor." In the first stage they often cry as much as they laugh, generally criticizing their own shortcomings. In the second stage, their hostile laughter is usually directed at others. By the third stage they no longer blame others for their problems and find the humor in their own inadequacies in a non-threatening manner. Once his patients reach the third stage, he says they no longer need treatment.

One expert recommends at least fifteen minutes of laughter a day. Here are some suggestions for helping the sufferer (and you) bring humor and laughter into daily life:

- Read humorous books.
- Watch comedy TV shows and rent comedy videos.
- Observe the humor in life's absurdities.
- Find comic relief in the local newspaper.
- Start a humor scrapbook or bulletin board of your favorite cartoons or humorous sayings.
- Share your sense of humor; reminisce about happy or funny incidents from the past.
- Romp with the kids; their silliness provides comic relief.
- Give yourself permission to be silly and find ways to add humor to the serious side of life.

While in the beginning the last thing the sufferer may want is humor, once recovery has started and this person has accepted his or her disorder, laughter can foster a recuperative atmosphere and provide some perspective on the problem.

Adding exercise, proper nutrition, and humor to the other recovery techniques will aid you and the sufferer in your battle against agoraphobia and panic disorder.

# A Meeting of the Minds: Mapping Successful Recovery Plans Together

*"It is not enough to take steps which may some day lead to a goal; each step must be itself a goal and a step likewise"*

*—Goethe*

Start the recovery process by making a recovery plan, setting recovery goals, and drawing up an agreed-upon "contract for success" through discussion, negotiation, collaboration, and agreement. You can write this recovery plan yourself, or you can obtain the guidance of a professional who specializes in agoraphobia and panic disorder.

This process says to the sufferer, "Yes, we recognize the problem exists and are willing to work together as a team to overcome it." This assures the sufferer that the team considers his or her problem a medical disorder, that it is out of the sufferer's control, and that the team cares enough to assist with recovery.

## ESTABLISHING A RECOVERY PLAN

Choose a meeting place where you can talk freely, and allow enough time for a complete discussion.

At the first recovery meeting, have the sufferer give you an account of his or her condition by asking the following questions: What are you afraid of? What causes you phobic anxiety? The sufferer must be as specific as possible.

If your loved one is afraid of more than one thing, ask him or her to list all of them. Ask, What happens to you when you are faced with the anxiety-producing situation? What do you feel and think, and what does it do to you? When did this condition first begin? What happened? The more you understand the problem, the more you can help.

Discourage the sufferer from discussing other problems and difficulties in his or her life, such as job or family problems. Also, don't allow the sufferer to analyze *what* caused the problem in the first place. Both of these distract from the overall goal.

Now you need to decide on a recovery technique. To do this, review what you already know about the disorder and possible methods of treatment (detailed in Chapter 4). The choice depends on the sufferer's recovery needs and financial ability.

Describe any emotional, financial, practical, or other benefits that you believe recovery will bring. Discuss how you can help the sufferer recover. Let the sufferer know you expect to make a commitment and play an active role in recovery. Tell him or her that you will be non-judgmental and understanding. While you can make suggestions about which recovery method to choose, the sufferer should always make the final decision.

In this session you must understand what the sufferer expects from his or her support persons during practice sessions. For instance, should the support people be quiet or talk during sessions when practicing facing fears? Make small talk? Remind the sufferer of what can be done to remain calm? Ask if the sufferer is feeling anxious?

In sessions, should support people stay next to the sufferer or walk behind him or her? Should they wait inside by the exit or outside in the car?

Ask the sufferer to make a list of do's and don'ts for practice sessions. Insist he or she be specific.

Once you have decided on a method of treatment and the sufferer has completed his or her list of do's and don'ts, set up another mutually convenient date and time for your next encounter. You will need a pencil and notebook for this session.

## THE SECOND MEETING: SETTING UP LONG-RANGE RECOVERY GOALS

### Establishing Recovery Goals

At this meeting, discuss what the sufferer wants to accomplish from recovery. Be more specific than "I want to get well." The sufferer might say, for example, "I want to be able to go places without being anxious and fearful, just as I could before my disorder. I want to drive to the store, across town, on freeways, in heavy traffic, over bridges, to the next city, and so on without being afraid or having a panic attack. I would like to go to the show or church again and do my own grocery shopping. I would like to drive my children to school or to soccer practice and play golf with my husband. I would like to fly someplace for vacation." Write these goals down in a notebook.

Next ask the sufferer to go over these written desires and narrow them down, setting specific priorities. What does he or she feel is most important at the present time?

For instance, does he or she want to be able to drive to the grocery store, or to just to shop there? Drive on the freeways, or drive the kids to school? Just leave the house? This process helps the sufferer identify long-range goals and decide which ones have priority.

Setting goals is an essential step that leads to change. Goals play an important role in overcoming agoraphobia and panic disorder.

### How to Set Long-Range Recovery Goals

The following guidelines and procedures, used by many recovery groups, will help the sufferer set his or her long-range recovery goals. These goals must be ones the sufferer wants to reach, not goals the support people think should be attained.

On a single sheet of paper write down the long-range recovery goals the sufferer wants to achieve. Be specific. Reducing anxiety to a minimal level is desirable, but as a goal this is too broad. Instead the sufferer might say, "I want to be able to go grocery shopping alone," "I want to be able to take my children to school," or "I want to be able to drive by myself on the freeway."

Next, on a page in your notebook, write the heading "Long-Range Recovery Goals." Under this heading copy your list of long-range goals. List the most important goal first and so forth.

# THE THIRD MEETING: HELPING THE SUFFERER SET SHORT-RANGE GOALS

## The ABCs of Setting Short-Range Goals

A. Create a notebook heading titled "Short-Term Goals."

B. Under this heading, write the number-one goal from the list of long-range goals.

C. Through brainstorming, modify this long-range goal into a more specific goal. For example, say the sufferer's top long-range goal is to be able to shop in the grocery store alone. Modify this long-range goal to the more specific "being able to buy four items in the grocery store by oneself."

D. Break down this *modified* goal into smaller goals that will lead to achieving the larger goal. List these smaller goals in subsequent order underneath the modified goal. For example:

*Long-Range Goal:* Shopping in the grocery store alone.
*Modified Goal:* Buying four items in the grocery store by oneself.
*Short-Range Goals:*
1. With your support person, sit in the parking lot looking at the grocery store.
2. Walk to the entrance with your support person, standing outside for 1-5 minutes, watching people go in and out.
3. Walk in and out of the store with your support person.
4. With your support person waiting outside the door, walk in and out of the store alone.
5. Repeat steps three and four, waiting inside for 1-2 minutes

instead of leaving immediately.

6. Enter the store with your support person and walk to the back of the store, staying there for 1-5 minutes.

7. Repeat step six several times, staying in the back of the store a little longer each time.

8. With your support person, remain in the store, browsing in different areas for 5-10 minutes.

9. Go into the store with your support person, buy one item, going through the quick-check line.

10. Repeat step 9 several times, buying more items each time until you've bought four.

11. With your support person waiting inside by the exit, buy 1-4 items, going through the quick-check line.

12. While your support person again waits in the car, go shopping by yourself. Repeat this step several times, gradually buying more items until you've purchased four and spent more time in the grocery store alone.

13. With your support person waiting at home by the telephone if needed, go to the store alone and buy four items. Repeat this step several times until you feel comfortable.

When the short-range goals are accomplished, the original long-range goal is then modified into more short-range goals until this original goal of shopping alone is achieved. For example, the last goal, Step 13, would then become the number-one goal on the next list of short-range goals, except perhaps the sufferer would buy five or more items. The sufferer's new list of short-range goals would include gradually buying more items and spending more time in the grocery store. Each step on the new list would then be repeated by the sufferer until this person could comfortably shop alone without the support person even waiting by the telephone.

Each time the sufferer accomplishes a long-range goal, he or she progresses to a new one, referring to the list of long-range goals. You and the sufferer then meet again to modify and break down the new long-range goal into smaller short-range goals to practice on. Always write them in a notebook.

When you have helped the sufferer define and write out the first short-range goals taken from the number-one long-range goal, you will have mapped out the first step in your recovery plan. (Additional sample "hierarchies" are included later in this book.)

## Elements Necessary to Successfully Achieve Goals

Dr. Hardy believed that certain processes are required for sufferers to be successful with recovery goals:
1. Know what you want to accomplish.
2. Define goals clearly.
3. Break goals into small, manageable steps.
4. Progress one step at a time.
5. Practice daily, or at least three times a week, 90 minutes a session. Research shows this is the optimal practice time. However, do not expect the sufferer to practice 90 minutes in the beginning.
6. Schedule practice times and commit to following that schedule.
7. Keep goal charts, along with a daily journal.
8. Reward accomplished goals.
9. Continue working on goals even when discouraged.
10. Recognize when the sufferer has reverted to old behavior patterns, then recommit to achieving the goal.

# TYPES OF RECOVERY GOALS

Because recovery techniques include a multitude of elements, the sufferer will recover easier and have a more solid foundation if he or she also includes the following goals:

## Behavioral

· Increase the mental ability to cope with anxiety producing situations. This includes the ability to do more things and be in more places without experiencing anxious reactions.
· Reduce the time spent worrying, as well as feeling guilty and ashamed.
· Learn communication and assertiveness skills. Sufferers need to let others know their likes and dislikes and what they do and do not want and need.

## Cognitive

· Mentally relax and recognize what triggers anxious reactions. Internal triggers include thoughts, beliefs, attitudes and bodily feelings.
· Overcome the belief that sufferers are helpless or that something is fundamentally wrong with them.
· Cultivate inner freedom and extinguish learned reactions.
· Overcome destructive and negative ways of thinking such as "all or nothing," "either-or," "what-if's," and so on.
· Accept and nurture yourself and overcome the unrealistic need for other's approval and affection.
· Realize that disagreement and criticism of others will not endanger existence.
· Overcome the fear of revealing the disorder (the fear of what people think).

## Physical

· Increase the body's ability to relax and the length of time the body can remain in a physically relaxed state.
· Increase the ability to replace physiological arousal with physical relaxation.
· Increase the time the sufferer can stay in the anxiety-producing situation.

## Philosophical

· Accept the responsibility for mental and physical well-being, as well as responsibility for the disorder.
· Find self-contentment and self-acceptance.
· Live for the present; take time to freely and completely enjoy life by doing things that will enrich it.
· Help other sufferers.

## KEEPING A RECOVERY GOAL CHART

A recovery goal chart offers a visual record of the recovery progress that often seems painfully slow.

This is not mandatory, but it can be extremely helpful. If you decide to use a goal chart in the recovery process, the goals should be short-term and limited to no more than twelve to fifteen steps. This visual record is a reminder that the more the sufferer practices goals, the more improvement he or she will make. Many teams also like to keep written records. (See Figure 6 for sample goal chart, Figure 7 for written records.)

## THE THIRD MEETING: ESTABLISHING A CONTRACT FOR SUCCESS

A contract for success between the sufferer and team members strengthens the recovery plan. This is the topic of the third meeting.

**Figure 6. The Recovery Goal Chart.**

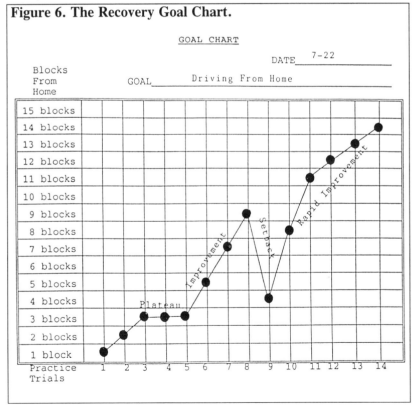

# Figure 7. Written Log for Goal Chart.

LOG FOR GOAL CHART

DATE____7-22_____                    GOAL_____Driving From Home_____

Trial

#1  With support person drove one block from home and came back, had #2 anxiety level, took 3 minutes to recover, tried again.

#2  With s/p drove two blocks from home and came back, had #2 anxiety level, took 3 minutes to recover, tried again.

#3  With s/p drove three blocks from home and came back, had #3 anxiety level, took 5 minutes to recover, tried again.

#4  With s/p drove three blocks from home and came back, had #3 anxiety level, took 4 minutes to recover, tried again.

#5  With s/p drove three blocks again and came back, had a #2 anxiety level, took 3 minutes to recover, tried again.

#6  With s/p drove five blocks from home and came back, had a little anxiety but no phobic reaction, tried again in four minutes.

#7  With s/p drove seven blocks from home and came back, had twinge of anxiety but again no phobic reaction, tried again in four minutes.

#8  With s/p drove nine blocks from home and came back, again had little anxiety, tried again in three minutes.

#9  With s/p drove four blocks from home and came back, faced more traffic, had #5 anxiety level, causing a setback.  Felt exhausted, decided had enough practice for the day.

DATE____7-24_____

#10  With s/p drove eight blocks from home and came back, had little anxiety and no phobic reaction, tried again in three minutes.

#11  With s/p drove eleven blocks from home and came back, again had no phobic reaction, tried again in two minutes.

DATE____7-25_____

#12  With s/p drove twelve blocks from home, then drove around in area a little and came back, had little anxiety, tried again.

#13  With s/p drove thirteen blocks from home, drove around a little and came back, had no anxiety, tried again.

#14  With s/p drove fourteen blocks from home, drove around again and came back, had no anxiety. Will start new goal chart.

A contract for success identifies the support people's roles along with their responsibilities and obligations. An agreed-upon contract with scheduled practice times is a useful guide and helps create discipline. Otherwise, everyday concerns tend to get in the way of consistently working on curing the disorder. Working on recovery needs to be a top priority.

Your contract for success can be verbal or written. A written agreement eliminates arguments over what was said or agreed upon. This agreement should come from a mutual understanding of both your and the sufferer's feelings, needs, and goals in relation to the recovery process.

I have included a sample contract for success that covers all the important elements needed. This agreement can be used as it stands or as a guideline from which to draw up your own personalized contract. Take a few minutes to read the contract and jot down on paper anything else you can think of that might benefit recovery. If you are concerned about a particular issue, make that a part of the recovery contract.

Consider how much time each of you can afford and are willing to commit to practice sessions. Remember, the more the sufferer practices, the faster he or she will recover. While regular practice takes self-discipline on the sufferer's part, Dr. Hardy found it important to work on some recovery goal every day. Only by regular, consistent practice will the sufferer make progress. Dr. Hardy suggested, at the beginning of each week, setting a specific time to practice every day of that week. The sufferer doesn't need to accomplish something every day, but the sufferer must at least take some daily action toward recovery.

# OUR RECOVERY CONTRACT FOR SUCCESS

## Part I: Support Person's Section

I, _____, as the main support person for _____, agree to do my best to make his/her recovery process successful by affirming the following statements:

1. I will make the following contract with my partner, and I am

ready and willing to do whatever work is needed to help.

2. I am committed to making recovery "our problem," not just my partner's problem alone. And I will help to create a "phobic nest" for him/her.

3. I will help my partner to find a self-help method or professional help, and I will attend all sessions necessary and read all the materials given.

4. To the best of my ability I will follow the guidelines for being a good recovery support person. And I will practice good communication and collaboration/negotiation skills to enhance the recovery process and my relationship with my partner.

5. I will remain with my partner in his/her recovery endeavor as long as he/she continues to try to recover, regardless of how long it takes.

6. I will do whatever I can to better understand my partner and the causes of his/her condition. I will try to tolerate, express, and encourage my own and my partner's feelings and fears; and do my best to be more open.

7. I will become educated about my partner's disorder, by reading information on it and learning all I can.

8. I will help my partner to practice facing fears through "no demand" practice sessions; following times stated in the contract addendum. I will learn to know my partner's stimulus trigger points (what sets off his/her anxiety) and help him/her to recognize them.

9. I will help my partner to set recovery goals, solve problems, negotiate difficulties and overcome setbacks; helping this person through the rough spots in his/her life.

10. I will do my best to discontinue criticism and help my partner to have a positive attitude; instilling a "You can recover" outlook.

11. I will do my best to make my partner feel emotionally, maritally, and financially secure. There will be no threats or discussion of separation or divorce. If my partner has problems that are interfering in his/her overcoming the disorder, I will welcome this person getting professional help for these issues and be willing to attend also, if needed.

12. I will welcome my partner taking control of his/her own

life and becoming more self-sufficient and independent. And I will set personal limits as to how much help is too much help, trying not to hold my partner's recovery back by being too solicitous.

13. I will welcome my partner joining a support group of his/her peers and making friends. If possible, I will also join a support group, making friends and learning from it as much as I can about how to be of help.

14. I will take pride in the fact that I helped expand my partner's world. And I will help him/her to continue to expand it by joining together with this person in social activities and by us making plans to go places and take trips together.

## Part II: Sufferer's Section

I,_____, as the person who suffers from agoraphobia and/or panic disorder, agree to do my best to make my recovery process successful, working together with _____, my support person, by affirming the following statements:

1. I will make the following contract with my partner, and I am ready and willing to do whatever work is needed to help myself recover, employing all the necessary recovery tools.

2. I will try my best to find a self-help method or professional help, and I will attend all sessions necessary, read all the materials given and complete any homework. To the best of my ability I will follow all the recovery guidelines necessary to overcome my disorder and I will make a firm commitment to the recovery process.

3. I will learn good communication and collaboration/negotiation skills to enhance my supported recovery process and my relationship with my spouse and/or support person.

4. I am willing to be responsible for my own disorder and for my recovery from that condition; trying my best to overcome this disorder, never giving up no matter how long it takes. If there are problems in my life that are interfering in my recovery, I will seek professional help, if possible. And, if needed, I will welcome my support person (spouse) attending, as well.

5. I will do whatever I can to better understand my support partner and his/her situation in relation to my disorder, including any

problems it causes this person. I will try to tolerate, express, and encourage my own and my support partner's feelings and fears; and do my best to be more open. And I will welcome my partner taking some needed time for himself/herself.

6. I will become educated about my disorder by reading information on it and learning all I can about its causes and the recovery process.

7. I will do my best to consistently practice facing my fears and anxiety through "no demand" practice sessions; following times stated in the contract addendum. I will learn my stimulus trigger points (what sets off my anxiety), and I will help my support partner to recognize them as well.

8. I will set recovery goals, and I will do my best to solve problems, negotiate difficulties and overcome setbacks.

9. I will do my best to overcome negative thinking and to have a more positive attitude, believing, "I can recover."

10. I will do my best to eventually take control of my own life and become more self-sufficient and independent. And I will set personal limits as to how much help is too much help, trying not to let my support partner take over and do too much for me.

11. If possible, I will join a support group of my fellow sufferers, making friends and learning from it as much as I can about how to recover. I will also welcome my support person joining a support group of his/her peers and making friends.

12. As I begin to recover, I will do my best to not stop recovery because I've reached a comfortable spot, but will work to continue expanding my world. When I am able, I will join in social activities, make plans to go places, even take trips together with my support person (spouse).

An addendum should be attached to your contract for success that states what each of you agree to do weekly toward recovery. This addendum needs to be periodically renewed and reevaluated as you move through different stages of recovery. Plan to meet at regular intervals—weekly before practice, bi-weekly, or monthly—to decide on future recovery steps. This is also a good time to discuss the past week and bring up concerns or questions. This meeting is a vital part of keeping the recovery process on the right track.

Always give the addendum a trial run to see if it works well. Then revise or modify it as needed. Any good agreement must be flexible, allowing for change and growth.

Here is a sample addendum:

I _____, agree to practice relaxation exercises twice daily. I also agree to do fieldwork with a support person ____ times per week for a period of ____ minutes a session.

I _____ , agree to provide quiet time for _____ by watching the children and answering the phone while he/she practices his/her relaxation exercises. I also agree to be available to help him/her with fieldwork ____ times per week for a period of ____ minutes a session.

Both sufferer and support person should remind each other that one doesn't have to be perfect as long as one sincerely aims for these ideals and makes some progress toward them.

Even if you decide not to use a detailed written contract, consider a written weekly agreement or at least a verbal agreement. This will help keep each of you disciplined.

When considering issues for the agreement, you should both allow yourselves time to think about your recovery wants and needs. Write them down. Then once your lists are complete go over them carefully, asking yourselves about each item. How important is this? How much does it mean to me and to recovery? Is this a realistic issue?

When you finally meet to discuss the contract and your separate lists, don't rush. And don't pretend to understand or agree with something if you don't. Ask questions; speak up. This is a good time to follow the collaboration/negotiation guidelines. Discuss each of your needs, wants, and goals for recovery. Be aware of your differences and settle them before you actually start working on the recovery steps. Discuss how each of you sees your future role in the recovery process. Also agree on your individual work requirements.

No matter how well designed, no agreement can make two people good recovery partners. You both must want the agreement to work.

*Chapter 11*

In the following chapter you will receive precise, detailed instructions about your role in the supported recovery process during practice sessions.

# Steering Clear of Fear: Putting Fieldwork into Action

*"Attempt easy tasks as if they were difficult, and difficult tasks as if they were easy: in the one case that confidence may not fall asleep, in the other that it may not be dismayed."*

—*Baltasar Gracian*, <u>The Art of Wordly Wisdom</u>

This chapter explains the how-to's of exposing the sufferer to feared situations using the in-vivo desensitization process. While the sufferer is serious about exposing him- or herself to this fear, realize that inside he or she is terrified. Here are some ways you can help before, during, and after exposure practice.

## BEFORE YOU BEGIN

· Make a photocopy of the anxiety scale (Figure 4) to take with you during exposure practice. This will help to monitor the sufferer's anxiety level. Also memorize Dr. Hardy's five Rs: react, retreat, relax, recover, repeat. If necessary, summarize what each means. Here is an example:

React: Confront fearful situations until the anxiety reaction is slightly
   uncomfortable, a #3 (or below) on the anxiety scale.
Retreat: Back away from the fearful situation. Walk toward the

door, take a few steps away, or turn around and face other way.

Relax: Distract mind and let self relax and calm down.

Recover: Completely recover from the anxious reaction.

Repeat: Approach the fearful situation again, repeating the five Rs process.

• Review the basics of support in Chapter 6 so they will be fresh in your mind. Use a notebook to start a practice diary that you and the sufferer can go over weekly. Record in it such things as the date, length of session, what was practiced, and how the session went. Note the problem areas and gold-star successes.

• Review the sufferer's list of do's and don'ts used for practice sessions. Also, make a plan for coping. Go over what the sufferer wants you to do when anxiety starts to rise or if he or she panics.

• Remind the sufferer that he or she must be willing to take risks and feel some discomfort, otherwise there will be little or no improvement. Dr. Hardy found that 40 percent of those who got stuck during recovery did so because they stayed too close to their safety zone.

• When arranging to meet somewhere during practice, decide ahead of time what to do if one of you misses the other. While being where you say you're going to be is important, there may be times when one or both of you will be unavoidably delayed.

• If the sufferer hesitates to face something previously decided upon, urge him or her try. Plan ahead what to do if he or she has difficulty. Also, don't pay close attention to failures.

• When the sufferer makes excuses for not practicing, be politely firm but insist he or she practice anyhow. If the sufferer refuses, drop it. You might say something like, "Okay, today may not be a good time, but we should try practicing again soon. You don't want to loose ground." Then suggest several possible practice times. Permit him or her to choose the date.

• When the sufferer's practice session entails attending some function, plan ahead how to leave if the sufferer has problems. It could be simply, "I'm not feeling well," or a special sign. The sufferer should never feel trapped.

· Have alternate plans closer to home when a practice session entails a trip. Then, even though the sufferer can't make it the full distance, he or she won't feel the exposure trip was a failure.

· Remind the sufferer that while he or she is practicing new recovery skills you are practicing new support skills. His or her role will take some trial and error practice; so will yours.

· Don't go into practice sessions with preconceived ideas of how far the sufferer can go. If you do and the sufferer falls short of set standards, he or she will feel like a failure. It's the attempt to practice that counts. Also realize that sometimes the sufferer can do more than at other times. Just because he or she could do something one day doesn't mean this person can do it next time.

· Prepare the sufferer before the practice session. Here are some thing you could say:

Remember, anticipation is always much worse than reality. It will be easier once we get started.

Remember, I will be here to help you use the techniques you have learned. And we will take things slowly, one step at a time.

You will be in total control of the situation at all times. And if you want to leave, we will.

Expect and allow that you may feel anxious and fearful, and if it happens, I will be there to help you. Expect and allow that fear and anxiety will disappear and reappear. And try to accept it when it does.

Remember, any tension you feel is a signal for you to use your coping techniques.

Label your fear according to the anxiety scale (from 1 to 10), so I will know how you are feeling.

Remember to keep your mind focused in the present.

You are going to do fine. I have confidence in you.

Remember this is just practice, not a demand situation. You do not have to do anything you don't want to do.

You don't have to be perfect. It's okay to make mistakes; treat them as learning experiences.

## HELPFUL HINTS

Avoid talking about the sufferer's feelings as much as possible. Instead, encourage interest in the surroundings: window displays, interesting people, clothes, furnishings, flowers. Keep the conversation pleasant, positive, and upbeat. Talk about things he or she is interested in.

Put your arm around the sufferer's shoulder when you approach the practice target. Squeeze his or her hand to help the sufferer remain in touch with the physical world, instead of allowing him or her to be overwhelmed by inner anxiety.

When you observe the sufferer breathing too rapidly, talking too fast, or hastily walking ahead, encourage him or her to slow down and behave in a calm, natural fashion.

Pay close attention to the sufferer's body movements and voice patterns—changes in speed or pitch can be signs of rising anxiety. Help the sufferer recognize early warning anxiety and panic signals by encouraging him or her to listen to what the body is saying.

Never push, and avoid overexposing or flooding. Always insist the sufferer retreat when the anxiety level reaches a #4 on the anxiety scale. Ignoring this can result in resensitizing the sufferer instead of desensitizing him or her to the fear being confronted.

When a planned practice session is successful, suggest that the sufferer attempt something a little more difficult. Sufferers can often do new things on impulse easier than they can carry out a planned agenda. Nudge, but if you get a "no," don't push.

Don't progress to a new goal too soon. This can lead to failure and discouragement. However, when it is necessary to repeat an individual goal more than a few times, consider making small changes each practice session. For example, if the goal is driving to the store, change from driving in the morning to driving in the afternoon, or change the route.

If the sufferer is frightened by strange feelings, help him or her refocus attention elsewhere. Since these feelings are symptoms of phobic fear, encourage the sufferer not to discuss them. Follow the same procedure as you would for a panic attack.

Let the sufferer know in advance that he or she can always leave fearful situations such as purchasing tickets to a movie. Reassure the sufferer its okay to leave anytime.

If the sufferer experiences anxiety, as long as it is not above a #3 level on the anxiety scale, try to encourage him or her to keep trying. If anxiety reaches a #4 or above, retreat. The desensitization process won't work because the sufferer's anxiety is too high.

## THINGS TO SAY DURING ANXIETY

If the sufferer prefers that you not talk during anxious periods, keep quiet and allow him or her to imagine being in the "safe place" and to concentrate on relaxing and proper breathing. Use a non-verbal message that says, "Everything is alright; I'm here for you."

Sometimes the sufferer will want you to talk to help him or her relax and refocus. Here are some things you can say:

Focus on where your body is tight and relax it there.

No matter how bad you feel, you can handle it. I have faith in you. They are just feelings and will not harm you.

Don't fight the feelings; accept them. Let them flow over you, everything will be fine soon.

Don't overwhelm yourself; take one thing at a time.

I know you can do it. (You've done it before.) Just tell me what you need me to do right now.

Everyone has fear sometimes. It is a normal feeling that rises; it will subside soon. Breath slowly from the abdomen, not the chest. Tell yourself you can cope. Think with your head, not with your symptoms.

Keep your mind in the present. Think about what you need to do. Stop worrying about the future.

Stop negative and scary thoughts now, and talk to yourself positively. Remember to use counterstatements.

Remember, it's your thoughts making and keeping you anxious, not the place you are.

Don't worry about what other people think. You'll probably never see them again, and they don't know you anyway.

## TO HELP COUNTER EARLY STAGES OF PANIC

Suggest the sufferer temporarily exit the situation until his or her anxiety subsides—go outside, step out of the checkout line, pull off the road.

Distract attention from the panic symptoms with simple repetitive activity—snap a rubber band on the wrist, count change, read license plates. Or do something focused such as working a jigsaw or crossword puzzle, counting backwards, reading a book or magazine, or playing cards. Do something physical to dissipate the anxious energy: take a short walk or work in the garden.

Suggest the sufferer get angry. One cannot be angry and anxious at the same time. Use some of the techniques for anger described earlier in the book: hit the bed with a rolled up newspaper, or pound a pillow. Suggest disrupting patterns of negative or fearful thinking using positive self-talk. Remind the sufferer to breath abdominally and to relax the muscles.

## WHAT TO DO ABOUT A PANIC ATTACK

Sometimes, no matter what you do, the sufferer will have a panic attack during a practice session. The sufferer will feel devastated, and you will feel helpless and unsure what to do. But the anxiety attack is temporary, it will always subside, and it will not harm the sufferer's mind or body. After it is over do the following:

1. Remain calm; any agitation will make matters worse. Don't

say, "Snap out of it." If possible, don't let the sufferer go home-
—this could increase avoidance in the future. Suggest that he or she
back away temporarily. Find some place to sit close to the area
where the anxiety began. Try not to leave until the anxiety has
started to recede.

2. Hold the sufferer's hand or put your arm around him or her.
Have this person take slow deep breaths with the lower abdomen instead of upper chest. Tell him or her to let go of the anxiety with
each breath out. Remind the sufferer that unpleasant bodily feelings
are not harmful and that it will be over soon. Anxiety subsides in
waves, so the sufferer may feel two or three ebbs of fear before becoming calm. Allow him or her to be emotional, shaky, or whatever.
Don't keep asking how he or she feels; this makes the anxiety worse.
Again, use distraction techniques.

3. Have the sufferer tell you when the anxiety subsides. When
they do, try to talk him or her into practicing just a little while longer—once a panic attack has occurred it is unlikely for it to come
back for a while. Staying in the surroundings makes it easier for the
sufferer to cope next time.

4. When the anxiety dissipates, encourage the sufferer to discuss the feelings, and try to help this person locate the panic attack's
cause.

## If the Sufferer Must Leave

Sometimes the sufferer may not be able to stay in a situation
long enough for his or her anxiety to dissipate. If so, leave the situation but arrange another practice session soon. The sooner the sufferer faces the fear, the less chance of this turning into a
setback—which could spread to other practice areas as well. If you
return another time and the sufferer must leave again, the practice
item may be too difficult. Back up and start with something easier or
move on to something different.

## What Not to Do During Practice

· Even if the sufferer fails, never show open disappointment.

- Never show that you are mad or frustrated; hold your temper. This includes non-verbal messages like disgusted looks or heavy sighs which could be interpreted as a "not again" attitude. And never be argumentative, as it will instantly bring on anxiety.
- Never trap the sufferer in a situation he or she doesn't want to be in.
- Just because the sufferer did well on one goal, never assume he or she can go further. Forcing can turn the relaxed feelings of success into panic and feelings of failure.
- Never avoid the sufferer when this person tells you he or she is anxious.
- Never use force.

## WHAT TO DO AFTER PRACTICE

Never forget to compliment and praise the sufferer on his or her success (even if minor). Praise also for genuine effort to try, even if he or she failed.

After each practice session ask the sufferer how he or she feels it went and continue to do this even when the sufferer starts practicing alone. Remain positive and avoid criticism. Expect the sufferer to sometimes feel exhausted after practice. This is normal.

Always take the sufferer right home after practice unless you ask first and he or she agrees.

## MAINTAINING REGULAR PRACTICE SESSIONS

Regular practice is vital to recovery, but when to push the sufferer and when to back off is the question I get asked the most. Dr. Hardy said no one can tell support people *how* to push and *when* to push; it is purely a judgement call on their part. When you push and you begin to get heavy resistance from the sufferer, back off. When you back off and the sufferer doesn't do anything, then push. If the sufferer isn't practicing, negotiate with this person. "Well, you haven't been practicing, so you're not making any progress and you're not getting any better. We need to practice and I'm willing to practice with you. Let's sit down and decide how we're going to do it. We'll make a plan and then we'll stick to that plan." Dr. Hardy recommended using the negotiation process, so when you and the sufferer start negotiating with one another you don't end up arguing.

# PRACTICE SUGGESTIONS

Along with the regular items the sufferer needs to practice, there are other ways to get out into the world to face fears.

• Rather than have things the sufferer wants to buy mail-ordered to the house, arrange to take him or her out to purchase these items, using shopping trips as practice sessions.

• Encourage the sufferer to visit friends and to make appointments with the hairdresser, dentist, or doctor. Let him or her know you will arrange an "out" ahead of time. Do this by telling these people in advance that he or she may not feel well and have to leave.

• Suggest the sufferer do volunteer work, join a club, or take a part-time job. These activities increase social capabilities and build self-esteem and confidence.

## Common Hierarchies/Practice Situations

See the hierarchy example for shopping in the grocery store in Chapter 11 and use this for practicing in any store. Always choose a time when the store is least busy.

Four other common hierarchies follow. Each are arranged in order of difficulty using graduated steps. Realize that these are just a structural framework to help reach the goal. For the hierarchy to be successful, the sufferer and the support person must use the recovery tools and techniques. When constructing your own hierarchies, take what you need from these suggestions, add to them, or leave out parts. Most need to be modified to meet each sufferer's special needs.

### Driving a Car

1. With sufferer at the wheel, sit in the car for a few minutes.
2. Have the sufferer drive one block on a quiet residential

street. Stops and starts should be slow and smooth.

3. Increase Step 2 to five blocks or more. Have him or her make right or left turns.

4. Have the sufferer drive on a street with a stop sign.

5. On a street with a minor traffic light, have the sufferer drive in the right lane.

6. Repeat Step 4 with the sufferer driving in the left lane and making left turns.

7. Have the sufferer drive on the edge of a downtown business district with a major arterial.

8. During non–rush hour traffic, have the sufferer drive in the right lane of the downtown business district.

9. Repeat Step 7, and have the sufferer change lanes and make right, left, and U-turns.

10. Repeat Step 7 during rush hour.

11. Have the sufferer drive on the right lane of the freeway for one or two exits.

12. Repeat Step 10. Have the sufferer pass cars and change lanes.

13. Repeat Step 11, gradually increasing the number of exits. (When I started to drive freeways alone, I did so one exit at a time, starting with the exits that were closest together.)

When the sufferer is ready to practice alone, all these steps can be repeated with you following behind in another car. Then repeat with you sitting by the telephone. These same steps can be used to desensitize the sufferer when riding with a support person as a passenger.

*Restaurants*

When beginning, always pick a time when few people are around.

1. Drive around the outside of the target restaurant with the sufferer.

2. Sit in the restaurant parking lot for five minutes, watching people enter and exit.

3. Enter the restaurant with the sufferer. Stay there from thirty seconds to a couple of minutes, then leave. If the sufferer feels awkward, ask to look at the menu as an excuse.

4. Enter the restaurant with the sufferer and sit at the counter. Order something that you won't have to wait for and that need not be finished, such as a soda or a cup of coffee (decaffeinated). A self-service restaurant is even easier. If the sufferer has to exit quickly, repeat this step several times until he or she can wait for what has been ordered.

5. Enter the restaurant with the sufferer and sit at a table by the door. Again, order coffee or a soft drink.

6. Repeat Step 5, but order a small meal, so the sufferer can get used to waiting for service and staying longer.

7. Repeat Step 5 sitting at a table away from the door.

8. Repeat Step 6 sitting at a table away from the door.

9. Repeat Step 6 when the restaurant is more crowded.

10. While you wait at a designated spot—in the car, by the telephone, even at a different area of the restaurant—have the sufferer repeat steps 4–8 without you. This could be done first with the sufferer entering alone and the support person entering later.

*Elevators*

1. Go with the sufferer to the lobby of a fairly busy building and watch people getting on and off the elevator.

2. Find an elevator in a building that is not busy and, with the sufferer, approach the elevator, watch it for a few minutes, and leave.

3. Walk with the sufferer into the elevator; push the button so the door remains open and the elevator remains stationary. Wait a few seconds, then exit.

4. With the sufferer, ride up one floor.

5. With the sufferer, ride up two floors or more.

6. Have the sufferer repeat Step 3 alone, with you standing outside the elevator.

7. Ride up one floor on the elevator alone, get out, and wait for the sufferer. This person rides up one floor and meets you where

you are waiting in front of the elevator door. Ride down together.

8. Repeat Step 7 increasing from one floor to two, and so on.

9. With you waiting on ground floor, have the sufferer ride up one floor, exit, then ride back down.

10. Repeat Step 9, increasing the number of floors.

11. With no one waiting, the sufferer rides up one floor alone, then down.

12. Repeat Step 11, increasing number of floors.

*Bridges*

In the beginning, choose a time of day where the bridge has little traffic.

1. Driving the sufferer, approach a short, narrow bridge. Stop, walk around, and look at the bridge. Watch cars using it.

2. Repeat Step 1 with the sufferer driving you.

3. Driving the sufferer, drive back and forth across the bridge several times.

4. Repeat Step 3 with sufferer driving you.

5. If possible, walk across the bridge and wait on the other side for the sufferer to drive over to meet you. Then drive back together.

6. Have the sufferer drive across the bridge alone and you follow in your car.

7. Have the sufferer drive back and forth across the bridge alone several times while you wait at the starting point.

8. The sufferer drives back and forth across the bridge alone without you present until he or she feels comfortable.

9. Repeat steps 1–8 with a longer bridge, gradually progressing to longer and wider bridges.

There are some practice situations in which you can first model for the sufferer how to perform the practice goal. For instance, have the sufferer observe you riding up and down an escalator. Keep this in mind when designing hierarchies.

## When the Sufferer Practices Alone

As soon as possible, encourage the sufferer to practice some things alone. Start with small things such as walking or driving around the block. This will start him or her on the road to independence. When you do this, always be available by telephone until the sufferer says you are no longer needed. Impress on the sufferer that he or she must call upon reaching the destination. Sometimes the sufferer feels so good about successfully making a destination that he or she forgets to call the support person!

This book has provided all the recovery nuts and bolts. Using the coping skills and supported recovery techniques discussed, you are ready to support the sufferer in whatever treatment plan he or she chooses. While putting these skills together and putting them into action can be hard work, it can also be exciting and rewarding.

Dr. Hardy found in-vivo desensitization works best under the following conditions: (1) When a person is ready to do it, and that means (2) being prepared through education and understanding the principles of facing rather than avoiding the problem, and when the person is aware of his or her body reactions and the stimuli which arouse anxiety. (3) When there is a strong commitment to recovery. (4) When practice goals are practiced with an empathetic and experienced person who understands the process.

To help you successfully complete your recovery journey, in the following chapter I will discuss what to expect during the recovery process.

# What to Expect During the Recovery Journey

*"The only way to predict the future
is to have power to shape the future."*

—Eric Hoffer, *The Passionate State of Mind*

The recovery period is often a chaotic one. Sufferers change constantly during recovery because of such things as emotional breakthroughs, setbacks, fluctuations of agoraphobia, and changes in personality and lifestyle. Some recovery changes cause the main support person and others closely associated to change as well. Support people need to be aware of what changes to expect in both the sufferer and themselves and to be aware of common recovery problem areas and how to handle them.

This chapter also discusses the importance of support people developing patience, perseverance, and a positive attitude to help them deal with recovery ups and downs.

## EMOTIONAL BREAKTHROUGHS

As sufferers begin to face previously avoided fearful situations, various feelings begin to surface. The feelings that appear often help sufferers clearly understand puzzling past experiences. When the feelings subside the rational part of the person is freer to think clearly and perceive his or her life patterns more objectively. Dr. Hardy expressed it this way: "This is when they stumble onto a previously hidden meaning for their anxieties. While it is joyful to discover, it is also painful in its memory."

These feelings sometimes come out as an explosion of emotions that for years the sufferer hadn't been able to express. If the sufferer never cries, gets angry, or laughs, he or she may have crying spells or outbursts of anger or laughter. Dr. Hardy found some sufferers even experience strong sexual feelings, go on a rampage of shopping or traveling, or engage in some other activity previously hindered by fear.

Dr. Hardy referred to this process as an "emotional breakthrough," and he likened it to "bubbles appearing on the surface of water about to boil."

When sufferers practice desensitization, he explained, they start removing the blocks that built their phobias. As they break down the walls, they experience the emotions that originally caused them to avoid various stimuli. Sometimes this makes them think they are getting worse. Actually, it means they are getting better. "Anxiety," Dr. Hardy said, "replaces normal feelings, and as the person gets better, normal feelings replace anxiety."

If an emotional breakthrough occurs, remind your loved one (using good communication skills) that this is healthy and expected. Try to get the sufferer to discuss and understand what he or she is feeling—often sufferers have no idea what that is. Or suggest this person talk to a therapist. It is vital that the sufferer express these emotions. Once this person openly talks about the incident and begins to understand it, he or she begins to resolve and accept the issues involved, which lessens this person's crying, anger, or whatever.

"Be patient through the eruptions," Dr. Hardy stressed, "as they will balance out and you will begin to see a beautiful new person emerge—if you're a spouse, maybe the original one you married."

· · ·

Chapter 13

# SETBACKS

It is common for sufferers to have setbacks while recovering. No one recovers without having them. However, sufferers can't have a setback until they have made some recovery progress.

Setbacks are a warning that progress has halted and the person has reverted to some of his or her old phobic behavior. They let the sufferer know that he or she needs to make some alterations in his or her environment, habits, and patterns of responding.

The initial setback devastates sufferers. Often, because they have reverted to all-or-nothing thinking, they tend to believe the gains they worked so hard to achieve are gone forever. This decreases or removes their motivation to overcome the setback.

Help the sufferer understand that to move forward he or she needs to reestablish the newly learned habits and behavior patterns. Explain that while uncomfortable, setbacks are a necessary part of the healing process. Accepting the reality of the situation is the first step to overcoming it. Counter the sufferer's feelings of frustration and defeat by suggesting he or she look at the setback as a chance to pause and take stock. Realize that this person may use your attitude about the setback as a model for his or her own.

Next, help the sufferer identify what caused the setback. Do this by examining what is presently happening in the sufferer's life. Dr. Hardy found there is usually a combination of two or three traumatic emotional events. While a major event can create a setback, so can any change or minor occurrence that causes a negative reaction. Sometimes the eager sufferer oversteps his or her present ability, and this imbalance causes setbacks.

Dr. Hardy recommended asking such questions as "Is there a situation in your life that may be interfering in your improvement?" "Have you recently had some traumatic emotional experience that you have suppressed your feelings about?" "Have you bitten off more than you can chew or overloaded yourself?" "Are you trying to be too perfect or thinking negatively again?" "Are you avoiding problems rather than solving them?" "Are you resisting change because it's too difficult?" "Are you not following the recovery program because you've gotten lazy?" "Have you become too passive, hoping someone will fix your disorder for you?" "Are you hoping for a magic pill or miracle to come along and make you well, so you've stopped trying?" "Have you been faced with a difficult situation that caused you to revert to phobic thinking?" "Are you worrying about what other people think or want rather than taking charge of your own life and doing what you want?" "Do you need to alter or improve any of your relationships with other people?"

He also suggests having the sufferer make a list of all the events in his or her life, no matter how small, that have recently occurred. Look at each item separately to see if there are any problems he or she is ignoring. Identify his or her feelings about each issue, then choose the items that elicit the strongest emotional response. Write options for resolving these problems. Finally, try some of the options using trial and error. Do not expect perfection.

Overcoming a setback is a one-step-at-a-time process and can take from a few days to a few weeks or longer. However, it generally takes less time to regain lost ground than it takes to initially attain it. The key is not to delay. It took one man four months to drive to Dr. Leman's office. When he lost that ability, he went to work on the problem immediately and regained it within a week. If there are problems, back up and have the sufferer work on easier items. In accomplishing those, he or she rebuilds confidence.

"As the sufferer's successes accelerate," Dr. Hardy said, "his or her setbacks will become less intense and more infrequent. With each setback recovery he or she will surpass previous accomplishments." Successes will then become more permanent.

If you find the sufferer having difficulty after trying the above techniques, he or she may need to talk to a therapist or some other anxiety disorder professional.

## THE CHANGES THAT RECOVERY BRINGS

As Dr. Hardy explained, "Getting well depends on change. If there is no change, there is no improvement." When the sufferer begins to face fears and feelings, his or her anxiety and fears increase and fluctuate.

Yesterday's successes—driving on the freeway, eating lunch in a crowded restaurant—cannot be duplicated today. Instead of being happy about successes, the sufferer becomes afraid to reveal them for fear he or she will be expected to be fully functional. One day the sufferer is elated because he or she "forgets" to be anxious, yet the next day he or she feels frustrated and depressed.

New patterns of thinking and ways to behave also cause the sufferer to develop new responses to his or her close relationships, creating uneasiness in the spouse and other support people. People often wonder, "Will he or she need me now that he or she is recovering?" In the past they knew what to expect from this person, and now they are not so sure. Although they want the sufferer to recover, it's not uncommon for a part of them to yearn for the past life they shared with this person.

Sometimes the new desire to be independent can be almost self-contradictory. He or she doesn't like relying on support people but needs them to get further from home. While excited about being able to go places, the sufferer may still resent the fact that he or she needed the support person's help.

Sometimes the behavioral changes dramatically alter the lives of the sufferer and the support people. For instance, a sufferer who was quiet or passive may become assertive. Unfortunately, when first trying to do so, he or she often goes to the extreme of being aggressive, suddenly taking offense to everything support people say and do. As therapist Lyn Simms, a former Terrap–Menlo Park group leader, explained, "You may feel as if your phobic partner has regressed to the 'terrible two's,' complete with a renewed interest in the word *no!*"

Dr. Hardy said, "It is only natural for them to become a bit power-hungry after such a long time of being a 'doormat.' Bear with them, and it will gradually balance out."

Sufferers may no longer seek other people's approval or wish to be like others. They may become self-accepting, too, and may also accept others as they are.

As the sufferer stops needing the help of family, friends, and co-workers, those who were always needed may start to feel neglected. Husbands and children may find that a wife and mother who was eager to please and was always there for them is busy with outside activities. Sufferers who were accustomed to staying home are making new friends and meeting new people. They find they can be social for the first time in many years. Sometimes their significant other begins to feel left out and starts feeling threatened. The immediate family may also resent the sufferer's absence and make him or her feel guilty.

Irritated, a spouse may mumble, "What took this person so long to recover? Look at all the wasted years." A spouse may also feel depressed and confused: "Doesn't he or she love me as much as before?" This person may also become increasingly suspicious of the sufferer's new-found freedom. He or she may have outbursts of anger and accusations, "Are you seeing someone else?" Some spouses may start having psychosomatic illnesses or subtly undermine the sufferer's confidence to keep the sufferer at home.

If relatives pressure the sufferer enough, they can cause him or her to regress. For example, one California woman was making great recovery strides, but resentment from the family because of her new part-time job and other minor outside activities, caused her to quit her job, drop out of her recovery program, and revert back to her old phobic habits. The family balance was restored, but her fears and anxieties soon returned.

Sufferers are sometimes so excited with their new-found selves that they tend to overlook others' feelings. Recovering spouses may forget to leave notes or call.

### How to Handle Recovery Changes

You and the sufferer should communicate about changes using the communication skills discussed in Chapter 9—phrasing your messages with "I" statements, and so on. Pay attention to your feelings; don't deny them. While these feelings may only be temporary, they can cause problems if not addressed.

Ask what the sufferer is feeling instead of taking the words at face value. Have patience with one another. Allow a period of adjustment while you learn to understand each other again. Fortunately, working together on recovery has put both of you in a good position to leave any old baggage behind.

"Give your partner the freedom to be independent," Dr. Hardy said, "by giving them the freedom to make mistakes and change, and they will give you the same courtesy in return."

If your relationship was unstable or unsatisfactory in the first place, it may get worse as the sufferer gets better. But if it has a good foundation, your relationship will improve as you work together in recovery.

While these times may be trying, if there are corresponding changes in both of you, the imbalance will only be temporary. If either of you find the difficulties more than you can handle, seek counseling together from a therapist who is proficient in anxiety disorders and family therapy.

Married couples grow stronger. Parents and children develop deeper affection and shared respect, friends become closer, developing an increased awareness of each other's needs—all because they became involved in the supported recovery process.

As Dr. Norman Vincent Peal once said, "Often what seem to be destructive adversities turn out to be creative assets, and those assets would not have become yours if something hadn't happened that at first seemed to ruin everything for you. Sometimes in poking around the wreckage you find your golden opportunity in what seems to be ruin."

As the sufferer becomes more independent, devote the time and effort you previously spent helping the sufferer pursuing your own activities. You have now developed patience, acceptance, perseverance, and unconditional love. Use these gifts to reach out to others. In doing so, you will find they will come back two-fold.

## TROUBLESHOOTING COMMON PROBLEM AREAS

Here are some common recovery problems and suggestions for solving them. Since readiness to recover can sometimes be at the root of many common problem areas, also refer to "Personal Factors and Secondary Gains" in Chapter 4.

·   ·   ·

## Excuses

While making excuses is a sign of avoidance, excuses are expected. Excuses often mean the sufferer's fear is so high he or she feels incapable of approaching this fear. "Whatever excuses the sufferer makes for not facing fears," Dr. Hardy said, "come solely out of fear of having an anxiety attack and *not* because he or she doesn't want to get well. If you can understand and really believe this, you will automatically be of more help than you know." Remind the sufferer that it's the accomplishment itself that counts, not the size of it. The euphoria that follows success motivates the sufferer to continue working on recovery.

## Resistance

Expect resistance in the beginning. This is often the first thing that happens in recovery. He or she is still operating under the negative habit of avoidance behavior. One problem is trying to set too high a goal. For instance, a sufferer may attempt to buy something in a grocery store the first time out, instead of just getting use to being there. As Dr. Hardy said, "If the goal is set too high, it will seem impossible and the sufferer won't try."

## Lack of Commitment

The recovery process is tedious. Sometimes the sufferer starts out fully committed to recovery only to lose interest and become discouraged. Unfortunately, the body cannot instantly unlearn the habits developed over a lifetime. Remind the sufferer that if he or she does not remain committed, he or she will revert to old behavior patterns. Also, make sure the goals set are based on what this person wants to achieve, not what others want.

## Discounting Success

The sufferer often sees practice sessions as either a complete success or a total failure. For instance, the sufferer wanted to drive ten miles on the freeway but could only drive two freeway exits, so he or she becomes upset. Point out that in the beginning, he or she couldn't even drive on the freeway at all, but eventually he or she will drive ten miles and more.

## Depression

Depression often leaves support people feeling hopeless. Blaming the sufferer, however, only aggravates the anxiety disorder. Handle depression by accepting it. Allow the sufferer to feel depressed. Encourage him or her to get out of bed and get dressed every morning even though he or she isn't going anywhere. However, also encourage sufficient rest. Remain positive about his or her treatment for depression and encourage the sufferer to stay with it.

## Lack of Progress

Some sufferers make little progress despite regular practice of hierarchies tailored to specific fears. This is usually caused from maintaining self-defeating thoughts and feelings about oneself or from relationship problems. If either of these is a problem, seek professional assistance from an anxiety disorder therapist.

## Low Motivation

Some sufferers want to recover but just can't get themselves motivated to practice. Or they start out very motivated but lose motivation once recovery slows. Here are some tips to increase practice motivation: (1) Make sure the practice method is appropriate for the sufferer's specific problems. (2) Set goals that are the proper size, and keep a goal chart so he or she can see progress. (3) Maintain a reward system that helps to outweigh the anxiety, such as a special gift for each goal reached. (4) Encourage the sufferer to talk about progress not only to you but to other people not directly affected by this progress, such as to fellow sufferers or by writing to an anxiety disorder newsletter. (5) Suggest the sufferer focus on increasing his or her performance rather than on decreasing the anxiety.

. . .

# PATIENCE, PERSEVERANCE, AND POSITIVE ATTITUDE

Support people often become discouraged with recovery and the changes it brings. Deal positively with all problems. Negative thoughts and actions bring negative results, affecting everything around you, including the sufferer.

If you work at being positive, even in the face of adversities, you will set the forces of faith, hope, and optimism in motion, and the sufferer will follow your lead. Experiment with different ways to lift your mood until you find something that works for you.

I read a few pages from a book on positive thinking each night and copied appropriately inspirational passages. This ingrained them in my mind and played a big part in changing my negative attitude. My husband and I also took recovery one day at a time. Self-talk and affirmations can be beneficial tools for support people, too.

If you are having a difficult time coping with recovery, review the methods of self-support in Chapter 7. And if you are experiencing difficulty with your support person role, talk it over with the sufferer's therapist.

Remind yourself and your loved one that getting good recovery results requires time, patience, persistence, and the will and fortitude to never give up. If you maintain a positive attitude and apply these three Ds—determination, dedication, and discipline to recovery—you can't help but be successful.

When the going gets tough, do what Norman Vincent Peale does; think of this old proverb: "The hammer shatters glass but forges steel. If you are made of good stuff, then the tough breaks will not break you but will make you hard like steel."

# Afterward: A New Beginning

*"The world is round and the place which may
seem like the end may also be only the beginning."*

—*Ivy Baker Priest, Parade*

By now you realize what a big difference you and others close
to the sufferer can make in recovery. By becoming involved, you decrease the chances of a relapse and speed recovery. You also have a
greater understanding of one another's position in relation to agoraphobia and panic disorder.

I urge you and the sufferer to reread this book and highlight,
with separate colored markers, any areas that are important to each
of you. Then go back over one another's.

All the recovery advice in this book can be summed up in one
sentence: Face the fear, and the fear will disappear. Just as you and
the sufferer have learned to live with his or her anxiety and fear, together you can learn to live a much more fulfilling life without it.

Recovery is a state of always becoming. It is a process of
growth and improvement that goes on for the rest of the sufferer's
life. Even after the sufferer completes recovery treatment he or she
needs to continue using and practicing recovery techniques in order
to move forward and preserve progress.

Throughout recovery never forget what you now know about
the type of people who are likely to suffer from agoraphobia with
panic disorder. Remember, they are highly sensitive and emotional.

They easily react to certain stimuli. They must express their feelings before they get too intense. They are people pleasers and perfectionists, and their background contributed to their condition.

Especially remember that you must accept the sufferer for what he or she is and that sufferers must also accept themselves. Keep in mind that sufferers must learn to be more realistic about themselves and the world in general and that to do so they must counter false beliefs and cognitive distortions with positive self-talk.

Above all, remember that recovery takes patience, persistence, and practice. It is a one-day-at-a-time process that should not have set time limits.

As your loved one continually progresses and grows, remind him or her of all these things. Remind the sufferer how important it is to keep setting goals for continual growth. After I had conquered the world around me, I continued to set goals to increase the size of this world by traveling away from home—first by car, then by plane. I set new personal goals for achievement to help others recover, to go back to college, to write this book. And I'm still setting them.

The sufferer must not slip back into past negative ways, which may contribute to the problem. Pay attention to any early warning signs that problems are recurring. If you see the sufferer thinking phobically again, remind him or her of the recovery tools necessary to counteract this.

As the sufferer continues to recover, help this person expand his or her support system so he or she can learn to trust others. Encourage the sufferer to take local self-improvement courses, such as assertiveness training or positive thinking. Encourage him or her to pursue a new interest or get a part-time job. Each new thing he or she does builds self-confidence and self-esteem and helps him or her lead a normal life.

Be aware that some sufferers reach a recovery plateau, such as being able to work, and become content to remain in the new comfort zone, growing no further. While their lives are better, they still aren't living fully. If this occurs, remind him or her of what has been achieved and point out that he or she can accomplish even more.

The recovery journey will be a difficult but challenging time for both of you. But in meeting this challenge, you will both emerge stronger, happier, and better than before.

It has been very rewarding for me to see sufferers and their relatives (especially couples) reach recovery success together. I have seen the supported recovery process turn around the relationships between sufferers and spouses or parents. Instead of hindering their loved one's recovery, they helped it. I have seen relationships grow and become better than they were in the beginning. I know that like them, you and your loved one can also become a recovery success story.

The sooner you start, the sooner it will happen. As Denis Waitley said in *The Joy of Working,* "Time is an equal opportunity employer. Each human being has exactly the same number of hours and minutes in every day. Rich people can't buy more hours. Scientists can't invent new minutes. And you can't save time to spend it on another day. Even so, time is amazingly fair and forgiving. No matter how much time you've wasted in the past, you still have an entire tomorrow. Success depends upon using it wisely—by planning and setting priorities. The fact is, time is worth more than money, and by killing time, we are killing our own chances for success."

Since my own recovery I have devoted my life to helping others recover, and I would love to delight in your success. I would also like to hear about your recovery experiences, what problems you faced, what material from this book helped you the most, and what other information you would like to see in a future recovery support book. Please let me hear from you.

If you are a clinician who treats agoraphobia and panic disorder or are involved in a self-help group, I want to hear from you as well. Dr. DuPont once told me he considered this condition to be a disorder of "quality people." I have found it to also be a disorder *treated* by "quality people"—people who work as a united front against these and other anxiety disorders. You are providing a wonderful, well needed service. Thank you.

Please write to:
Karen P. Williams
P.O. Box 166
Rocklin, CA 95677

# Anxiety Disorder Newsletter Resources

Some newsletters provide pamphlets, booklets, video and audio tapes, and other valuable information for sale to the consumer.

*ADAA Reporter*, published by the Anxiety Disorder Association of America, 6000 Executive Blvd., Suite 513, Rockville, Maryland, 20852 -3801, (301) 231-9350.

*Network News,* for self-help groups, also published by the ADAA.

*TERRAP Times,* published by TERRAP, 932 Evelyn Avenue, Menlo Park, California, (415) 327-1312 or 1 (800) 2-PHOBIA.

*National Panic/Anxiety Disorder Newsletter,* NPAD, Inc. 1718 Burgundy Place, Suite B, Santa Rosa, California 95403 (707) 527-5738.

*Anxiety Newsletter,* The Anxiety & Phobia Treatment Center, P.O. Box 80181, Valley Forge, Pennsylvania 19484 (215) 783-6964.

# Bibliography

American Psychiatric Association. *Diagnosis and Treatment of Anxiety Disorders: A Physician's Handbook.* Washington, D.C.: American Psychiatric Press, 1989.

Anxiety Disorder Association of America. *PSA Newsletter* (now *ADAA Reporter*), vol. 8, no. 3, July 1989.

Bourne, E. J., Ph.D. *The Anxiety and Phobia Workbook.* Oakland, California: New Harbinger Publications, 1990.

Doctor, R. M., Ph.D., and Kahn, A. *The Encyclopedia of Phobias, Fears, and Anxieties.* New York: Facts on File, 1989.

DuPont, R. L., M.D. *Phobias and Panic.* Rockville, Maryland: The Phobia Society of America [now known as The Anxiety Disorder Association of America], 1986.

Goldstein, A., and Stainback, B. *Overcoming Agoraphobia.* New York: Viking Penguin, 1987.

Greist, J. H., M.D.; Jefferson, J. W., M.D.; and Marks, I. M., M.D. *Anxiety and Its Treatment.* Washington, D.C.: American Psychiatric Press, 1986.

Hardy, A. B. *Agoraphobia: Symptoms, Causes, and Treatment.* Menlo Park, California: TERRAP, 1984.

Hardy, A. B., and Falkowitz, L. *Everything You've Always Wanted to Know About Phobias . . . but Had No One to Ask.* Menlo Park, California: TSC Management Corporation, 1987.

Hardy, A. B., and Flaxman, N. J. *TERRAP Program Manual.* Menlo Park, California: TSC Management Corporation, 1986.

Lindemann, C., Ph.D., Ed. *Handbook of Phobia Therapy.* New

Jersey: Jason Aronson, 1989.

Marlin, E. *Relationships in Recovery*. New York: Harper & Row, 1990.

McCullough, C. J., and Mann, R. W. *Managing Your Anxiety*. Los Angeles: Jeremy P. Tarcher, 1985.

McGarrah, M., M.S.W. *Help Yourself: A Guide to Organizing a Phobia Self-Help Group*. Rockville, Maryland: The Anxiety Disorder Association of America, 1990.

McKay, M., Ph.D.; Davis, M., Ph.D.; and Fanning, P. *Messages*. Oakland, California: New Harbinger Publications, 1983.

Munjak, D. J. *A Consumer's Guide to Medications*. Rockville, Maryland: Anxiety Disorder Association of America.

Padus, E., and editors of *Prevention* magazine. *The Complete Guide to Your Emotions and Your Health*. Emmaus, Pennsylvania: Rodale Press, 1986.

Peter, L. J., and Dana, B. *The Laughter Prescription*. New York: Ballantine Books, 1982.

Univeristy of California , Berkeley. *Wellness Letter,* vol. 9, no. 1, October 1992.

University of California, Berkeley, *Wellness Letter* editors. *The Wellness Encyclopedia*. Boston: Houghton Mifflin, 1991.

Wilson, R. R. *Don't Panic: Taking Control of Anxiety Attacks*. New York: Harper & Row, 1986.

Woolis, R., M.F.C.C. *When Someone You Love Has a Mental Illness*. New York: Jeremy P. Tarcher/Perigee, 1992.

Zane, M. D., and Milt, H. *Your Phobia*. Washington, D.C.: American Psychiatric Press, 1985.